The Diabetic Man's Complete Guide to Erectile Health

Proven Strategies to Restore Sexual Confidence and Performance Naturally

I0212905

Mariatu Moseph Ngeno

Important Medical Disclaimer

The Diabetic Man's Complete Guide to Erectile Health: Proven Strategies to Restore Sexual Confidence and Performance Naturally is intended for educational and informational purposes only. This book is not intended to be a substitute for professional medical advice, diagnosis, or treatment.

Medical Advice Disclaimer

The information contained in this book is based on the author's research and experience and is intended to provide general information about diabetes-related erectile dysfunction. However:

- **This book does not constitute medical advice** and should not be used as a substitute for consultation with qualified healthcare professionals.

- **Individual results may vary** based on personal health conditions, medical history, and adherence to treatment protocols.

- **Always consult your physician** before starting, stopping, or modifying any medical treatment, medication, or lifestyle intervention described in this book.

- **Emergency situations** require immediate medical attention. If you experience any medical emergency, including priapism (erection lasting more than 4 hours), chest pain, or severe allergic reactions, seek immediate emergency medical care.

Treatment and Medication Disclaimer

- All treatment options, medications, and medical devices mentioned in this book should only be used under the supervision of qualified healthcare providers.

- The author does not prescribe medications or provide individualized medical recommendations.

- Medication dosages, side effects, and contraindications mentioned are for educational purposes only and may not apply to your specific situation.

- Insurance coverage information is general in nature and may not reflect your specific plan benefits.

Lifestyle and Dietary Information Disclaimer

- Dietary recommendations and exercise protocols should be reviewed with your healthcare provider before implementation, especially if you have diabetes, heart disease, or other medical conditions.

- Blood sugar monitoring protocols are general guidelines and should be individualized based on your specific medical needs and current treatment plan.

- The author is not a registered dietitian, and nutritional advice should be confirmed with qualified nutrition professionals.

Names and Identity Disclaimer

Case Studies and Examples

All case studies, patient examples, and personal stories presented in this book are either:

- **Composite examples** created from multiple real-world scenarios to illustrate common patterns and outcomes, or

- **Fictional scenarios** based on typical presentations and treatment responses, or

- **Real cases** where identifying details have been substantially modified to protect patient privacy.

No real patient names or identifying information have been used without explicit written consent. Any resemblance to actual persons, living or deceased, or actual medical cases is purely coincidental.

Healthcare Provider References

When healthcare providers, medical institutions, or specific doctors are mentioned:

- **General references** to medical specialties, treatment centers, or healthcare systems are for educational purposes only and do not constitute specific endorsements or recommendations.

- **Specific physician names** mentioned in research contexts refer to published medical literature and do not imply personal or professional relationships with the author.

- The author does not personally endorse or recommend specific healthcare providers unless explicitly stated.

Product and Service Mentions

References to specific medications, medical devices, healthcare services, or commercial products are included for educational purposes only and do not constitute endorsements unless explicitly stated. The author may not have personal experience with all products or services mentioned.

General Legal Disclaimer

Limitation of Liability

The author, Mariatu Moseph Ngeno, and the publisher shall not be held liable for any direct, indirect, incidental, special, or consequential damages arising from the use of information in this book, including but not limited to:

- Medical complications or adverse reactions

- Financial losses from treatment decisions

- Relationship or personal consequences

- Any other damages resulting from reliance on the information provided

No Guarantees

While the strategies and information presented in this book are based on current medical knowledge and research:

- **No guarantee** is made regarding specific health outcomes or treatment success

- **Individual results will vary** based on numerous personal and medical factors

- **Success stories** presented are not typical results and should not be expected by all readers

Professional Relationships Disclaimer

The author has endeavored to provide accurate and current information as of the publication date. However:

- Medical knowledge and treatment protocols continue to evolve

- New research may contradict or modify recommendations presented in this book

- Readers should seek current medical guidance for the most up-to-date treatment approaches

---

Informed Consent and Acknowledgment

By reading and using the information in this book, you acknowledge that:

1. You understand this book is for educational purposes only

2. You will consult with qualified healthcare providers before implementing any suggestions

3. You accept full responsibility for your health decisions and their consequences

4. You understand the limitations and disclaimers outlined above

---

Emergency Contact Information

In case of medical emergency, immediately contact:

- **Emergency Services: 911** (United States)

- **Poison Control: 1-800-222-1222** (United States)

- **National Suicide Prevention Lifeline: 988** (United States)

For non-emergency medical questions, always contact your healthcare provider first.

ISBN: 978-1-7642100-7-2

Isohan Publishing

Table of Contents

Chapter 1: The Hidden Epidemic

The statistics might shock you. Walk into any diabetes clinic, and three out of four men sitting in that waiting room will experience erectile dysfunction at some point in their journey with diabetes. That's not a medical anomaly—that's a predictable consequence of a disease that affects every blood vessel, nerve, and hormone in your body.

You're reading this book because something has changed. Maybe it started subtly—erections that weren't quite as firm, or took longer to achieve. Perhaps it hit you suddenly one night, leaving you confused and frustrated. Either way, you've likely felt isolated, embarrassed, and wondering if your sex life is over.

Let me be clear from the start: it's not.

Breaking the Silence

The numbers tell a story that most men never hear. Research consistently shows that between 35% and 90% of men with diabetes will experience erectile dysfunction, with most studies settling around the 75% mark. That means if you're dealing with this challenge, you're part of a massive, largely silent majority.

Consider these facts: Men with diabetes develop ED 10 to 15 years earlier than men without diabetes. They're three times more likely to experience erectile problems. And yet, fewer than 25% of men with diabetes-related ED ever discuss it with their healthcare providers.

Why the silence? The answer lies in a toxic mix of shame, misinformation, and the mistaken belief that ED is somehow a reflection of masculinity rather than a medical condition with clear biological causes.

Case Example 1: Marcus, Age 42

Marcus had been managing Type 2 diabetes for six years when he first noticed changes in his erections. A construction foreman with a 20-year marriage, he initially blamed stress from work. "I thought maybe I was just tired," he recalls. "The job was demanding, and I figured once things calmed down, everything would go back to normal."

But months passed, and instead of improving, his erectile function continued to decline. His wife Sarah began to worry that he was losing interest in her. Marcus started avoiding intimate situations altogether, creating distance in a marriage that had always been strong.

"I felt like less of a man," Marcus admits. "I'm supposed to be the provider, the strong one. How could I tell my wife that my body was failing me? How could I admit to my doctor that I couldn't perform the most basic male function?"

The breakthrough came during a routine diabetes appointment when his endocrinologist specifically asked about sexual function. "I was shocked that she brought it up," Marcus says. "I realized this wasn't some personal failure—it was part of my diabetes that needed medical attention just like my blood sugar."

Case Example 2: David, Age 58

David's story began differently. A recently retired accountant with well-controlled Type 1 diabetes for over 30 years, he experienced a sudden onset of ED following a period of stress and poor glucose control during his father's illness.

"I'd managed my diabetes well for decades," David explains. "My A1C was always in range, I exercised regularly, ate well. Then my father got sick, and for about six months, my diabetes management went out the window. I was stressed, eating poorly, not checking my blood sugar as often as I should have."

2

During this period, David noticed not just erectile problems but also some numbness in his feet—early signs of diabetic neuropathy. "It was a wake-up call that even someone who thought they had diabetes figured out could still face complications."

The good news for David was that addressing his blood sugar control and seeking treatment for ED led to significant improvement in both areas. "Getting my glucose back in range helped with the nerve issues, and the ED medications worked well once my overall health improved."

Case Example 3: James, Age 29

Perhaps the most challenging cases involve younger men like James, who was diagnosed with Type 2 diabetes at age 26 and began experiencing ED just three years later.

"I felt like my life was over before it really started," James says. "I was dating, trying to build a career, and suddenly I had this older man's disease affecting the most intimate part of my life."

James's case highlights how diabetes-related ED can affect men at any age, particularly when diabetes develops early or isn't well-controlled initially. His A1C at diagnosis was 11.2%—significantly elevated—and it took nearly two years to achieve good glucose control.

"The hardest part was dating," James reflects. "How do you explain to someone you're getting serious with that you might need medication or other help to have sex? I almost gave up on relationships entirely."

James's story has a positive trajectory. With excellent diabetes management, weight loss, regular exercise, and appropriate medical treatment for ED, his sexual function improved significantly. He's now married and credits his early experience with ED for motivating him to take exceptional care of his diabetes.

The Mind-Body Connection

These stories illustrate a crucial point: ED doesn't just affect your body—it impacts your entire life. Research indicates that 79-80% of men with ED experience associated anxiety and depression. This creates what researchers call the "performance anxiety cycle."

Here's how it works: You experience erectile difficulties, which creates anxiety about future sexual encounters. This anxiety releases stress hormones like cortisol and adrenaline, which actually interfere with the biological processes necessary for erections. The result? More erectile problems, more anxiety, and a downward spiral that can seem impossible to break.

The psychological impact extends beyond sexual performance. Men with untreated ED report:

- Decreased overall life satisfaction
- Increased rates of depression
- Relationship strain and conflict
- Social withdrawal and isolation
- Reduced self-confidence in non-sexual areas
- Increased risk of other health problems due to avoidance of medical care

But here's the encouraging news: treating ED doesn't just improve sexual function—it improves overall quality of life, relationship satisfaction, and even motivation to manage other health conditions like diabetes.

ED as Your Body's Early Warning System

One of the most important concepts you need to understand is that erectile dysfunction often serves as an early warning system for other health problems. The blood vessels in the penis are smaller than those in the heart, so vascular problems often show up as ED before they cause heart problems.

4

Research shows that men with ED are at significantly higher risk for:

- Heart attack (45% increased risk)
- Stroke (25% increased risk)
- Peripheral artery disease
- Worsening diabetes complications

This means that addressing your ED isn't just about improving your sex life—it's about protecting your overall health. Men who seek treatment for ED often discover other health issues that need attention, from undiagnosed heart disease to poorly controlled diabetes.

The cardiovascular connection is particularly strong. Studies show that symptoms of ED may precede a major cardiovascular event by up to five years. This gives you a window of opportunity to address both your sexual health and your heart health simultaneously.

The Cost of Silence

What happens when men don't seek help for diabetes-related ED? The consequences extend far beyond the bedroom:

Relationship Impact: Untreated ED strains even the strongest relationships. Partners may feel rejected, unattractive, or blame themselves for the problem. Communication breaks down, intimacy decreases, and some relationships don't survive the stress.

Health Consequences: Men with untreated ED are less likely to manage their diabetes well. They avoid doctor visits, skip medications, and neglect self-care. This leads to worse diabetes control and increased risk of complications.

Economic Costs: Poor diabetes management due to avoidance of medical care leads to more emergency room visits, hospitalizations, and expensive complications. The cost of treating advanced diabetes complications far exceeds the cost of addressing ED early.

Quality of Life: Perhaps most importantly, men with untreated ED report significantly lower quality of life scores across multiple domains—not just sexual satisfaction, but overall happiness, work performance, and social relationships.

Breaking Down Barriers to Treatment

The good news is that once men seek help, the outcomes are usually positive. Modern treatments for diabetes-related ED are effective, safe, and varied enough that virtually every man can find an approach that works for his situation.

The first barrier to break down is the shame barrier. ED is not a character flaw, a sign of weakness, or a reflection of your worth as a man. It's a medical condition with clear biological causes and effective treatments.

The second barrier is the communication barrier. Your healthcare providers need to know about your sexual health to help you effectively. Most providers won't ask unless you bring it up, not because they don't care, but because they want to respect your privacy.

The third barrier is the expectation barrier. ED treatment isn't about returning to the sexual function of a 20-year-old. It's about achieving satisfying sexual function within the context of your current health, age, and relationship.

Practical Tools

Self-Assessment Questionnaire (IIEF-5)

Rate each question on a scale of 1-5 (1 = almost never/never, 5 = almost always/always):

1. How confident are you that you could get and keep an erection?

2. When you had erections with sexual stimulation, how often were your erections hard enough for penetration?
3. During sexual intercourse, how often were you able to maintain your erection after penetration?
4. During sexual intercourse, how difficult was it to maintain your erection to completion?
5. When you attempted sexual intercourse, how often was it satisfactory for you?

Scoring: 22-25 = No ED; 17-21 = Mild ED; 12-16 = Mild to moderate ED; 8-11 = Moderate ED; 5-7 = Severe ED

"Am I Ready for Help?" Checklist

Check all that apply:

- ED has been present for more than 3 months
- ED is affecting my relationship
- I feel anxious or depressed about sexual performance
- I'm avoiding intimate situations
- My partner has expressed concern
- I'm interested in exploring treatment options
- I'm ready to discuss this with a healthcare provider

If you checked 3 or more items, you're ready to seek help.

Partner Discussion Preparation Guide

Before talking with your partner:

1. Choose a non-sexual time and private setting
2. Start with your feelings, not blame
3. Explain that ED is related to your diabetes
4. Emphasize that it's not about attraction or love
5. Ask for their support in seeking treatment
6. Discuss how you can maintain intimacy during treatment

Taking the First Step

The journey from isolation to treatment begins with a single step: acknowledging that ED is a medical condition that deserves medical attention. You wouldn't hesitate to seek treatment for high blood pressure or an injury. Your sexual health deserves the same consideration.

Modern medicine offers more treatment options for diabetes-related ED than ever before. From simple lifestyle changes to advanced medical treatments, there's an approach that can work for your situation, your budget, and your preferences.

The men whose stories we've shared—Marcus, David, and James—all found their way back to satisfying sexual function. Their journeys were different, their treatments were different, but they all shared one thing: they decided that their sexual health mattered enough to seek help.

You deserve the same opportunity for recovery and satisfaction. The first step is recognizing that you're not alone, you're not broken, and you're not beyond help.

Moving Forward

ED affects millions of men with diabetes, but it doesn't have to define your life or your relationships. With proper understanding, appropriate treatment, and the right support, most men with diabetes-related ED can achieve satisfying sexual function.

The next chapter will help you understand exactly how diabetes affects your sexual function. This knowledge isn't just academic—it's practical information that will help you work with your healthcare providers to develop the most effective treatment approach for your specific situation.

Key Takeaways:

- ED affects 75% of men with diabetes—you're part of a large, largely silent community

- ED is a medical condition with biological causes, not a personal failure
- Untreated ED affects relationships, health management, and overall quality of life
- ED can serve as an early warning system for cardiovascular problems
- Modern treatments are effective for most men with diabetes-related ED
- The first step to recovery is recognizing that sexual health deserves medical attention
- You're not alone, and with proper treatment, improvement is possible

Chapter 2: How Diabetes Affects Erections

Understanding how diabetes affects your sexual function isn't just medical curiosity—it's practical knowledge that will help you make informed decisions about treatment and give you realistic expectations about recovery. More importantly, it will help you recognize that what's happening to your body has clear, biological explanations that have nothing to do with your worth as a man.

The relationship between diabetes and erectile dysfunction isn't mysterious or complex when broken down into understandable terms. Think of your body as a sophisticated machine where multiple systems must work together for proper sexual function. Diabetes affects every one of these systems, but understanding how gives you power to address each issue systematically.

The Erection Process Explained

Before we can understand what goes wrong, we need to understand what goes right. A normal erection requires the coordination of four major body systems: vascular (blood vessels), neurological (nerves), hormonal (hormones), and psychological (mind).

The Blood Flow System

Your penis contains two cylindrical chambers called the corpora cavernosa. These chambers are filled with spongy tissue that has thousands of tiny blood vessels. During arousal, these blood vessels dilate (open up), allowing blood to flow in rapidly. At the same time, the veins that normally drain blood from the penis become compressed, trapping blood in the chambers and creating rigidity.

This process requires healthy blood vessels that can respond quickly to nerve signals. The blood vessels must be able to expand to allow increased blood flow, and the mechanism that traps blood must work efficiently.

The Nerve Communication System

Sexual arousal begins in the brain and travels through the spinal cord to the nerves that control penile blood flow. These nerves release chemical messengers (neurotransmitters) that signal the blood vessels to relax and expand.

This system requires intact nerve pathways from the brain to the penis, functioning nerve endings in penile tissue, and proper production and release of neurotransmitters.

The Hormonal System

Testosterone plays multiple roles in sexual function. It affects libido (sexual desire), supports the health of erectile tissue, and influences the sensitivity of nerves and blood vessels to arousal signals.

Other hormones, including insulin, also affect sexual function. Proper hormone balance is necessary for optimal sexual response.

The Psychological System

Sexual arousal begins in the brain. Stress, anxiety, depression, and other psychological factors can interfere with the signal pathways that initiate and maintain erections.

The psychological system both initiates sexual response and can interfere with it when problems develop.

Seven Ways Diabetes Disrupts Sexual Function

Diabetes affects every system necessary for healthy erectile function. Understanding these pathways helps explain why ED is so common in men with diabetes and why treatment often requires addressing multiple factors simultaneously.

1. Vascular Damage and Blood Flow Issues

High blood sugar damages blood vessels throughout the body, including the small arteries that supply the penis. This damage occurs through several mechanisms:

Endothelial dysfunction: The inner lining of blood vessels (endothelium) becomes less responsive to signals that normally cause vessel dilation. This makes it harder for blood vessels to open up during arousal.

Atherosclerosis: High blood sugar accelerates the formation of plaque in arteries, reducing blood flow to the penis.

Reduced nitric oxide production: Nitric oxide is the key chemical messenger that causes penile blood vessels to relax and expand. Diabetes reduces the production and effectiveness of nitric oxide.

Case Example: Robert, Age 55

Robert, a 55-year-old teacher with Type 2 diabetes for eight years, noticed that his erections were gradually becoming less firm over a two-year period. His A1C had been running between 8.5-9.0% during this time—well above the recommended 7.0%.

During his evaluation, Doppler ultrasound testing showed significant impairment in penile blood flow. His peak systolic velocity (a measure of arterial inflow) was 25 cm/sec, compared to the normal range of 35-40 cm/sec.

"I knew my blood sugar had been high, but I didn't realize it was affecting my circulation in that way," Robert explains. "When the doctor showed me the blood flow measurements, it made sense why the pills weren't working as well as they used to."

Robert's treatment focused first on improving his diabetes control through medication adjustments and lifestyle changes. Over six months, he achieved an A1C of 7.2%. Repeat blood flow testing showed improvement to 32 cm/sec, and his response to PDE5 inhibitors improved significantly.

2. Nerve Damage (Diabetic Neuropathy)

Diabetic neuropathy can affect the autonomic nerves that control erectile function. These nerves are responsible for transmitting arousal signals from the brain to the blood vessels in the penis.

Nerve damage from diabetes typically develops gradually and may affect:

Sensation: Reduced sensitivity in penile tissue can make arousal more difficult to achieve and maintain.

Autonomic function: Damage to autonomic nerves interferes with the automatic processes that control blood flow during erections.

Signal transmission: Even when nerves aren't completely damaged, high blood sugar can interfere with the transmission of nerve signals.

3. Hormonal Imbalances and Testosterone

Diabetes affects hormone production in several ways:

Direct testicular effects: High blood sugar can damage the cells in the testicles that produce testosterone.

Insulin resistance effects: Insulin resistance, common in Type 2 diabetes, can interfere with testosterone production and increase the conversion of testosterone to estrogen.

Stress hormone effects: Poor diabetes control increases cortisol levels, which can suppress testosterone production.

Weight-related effects: Obesity, common in Type 2 diabetes, leads to increased conversion of testosterone to estrogen in fat tissue.

Case Example: Michael, Age 48

Michael was diagnosed with Type 2 diabetes at age 45 and began experiencing both decreased libido and erectile dysfunction within two years. His initial evaluation revealed a testosterone level of 185 ng/dL (normal range 300-1000 ng/dL).

"I thought the diabetes medication was affecting my sex drive," Michael says. "I didn't realize that diabetes itself could lower testosterone."

Michael's treatment included both diabetes management and testosterone replacement therapy. His endocrinologist started him on testosterone gel while optimizing his diabetes medications and encouraging weight loss.

Over eight months, Michael lost 35 pounds, achieved an A1C of 6.8%, and his testosterone level improved to 450 ng/dL with replacement therapy. Both his libido and erectile function improved significantly.

"It wasn't just one thing," Michael reflects. "Getting my weight down, my blood sugar controlled, and my testosterone level normal all worked together."

4. Psychological Factors

The stress of managing a chronic disease like diabetes, combined with the anxiety about sexual performance, creates psychological barriers to sexual function.

Performance anxiety: Once ED occurs, anxiety about future sexual encounters can perpetuate the problem.

Depression: Men with diabetes have twice the risk of depression compared to men without diabetes. Depression commonly affects libido and sexual function.

Stress: Chronic stress from diabetes management, work, and relationships increases cortisol levels and interferes with sexual response.

Body image issues: Changes in weight, energy, or physical capabilities related to diabetes can affect sexual confidence.

5. Medication Side Effects

Many medications used to treat diabetes and its complications can affect sexual function:

Blood pressure medications: Some beta-blockers and diuretics can reduce blood flow to the penis or interfere with nerve signals.

Antidepressants: SSRIs and other antidepressants commonly cause sexual side effects.

Other diabetes medications: While most diabetes medications don't directly cause ED, some individuals may be sensitive to certain drugs.

6. Inflammation and Oxidative Stress

High blood sugar creates chronic inflammation and oxidative stress throughout the body, including in erectile tissue.

Inflammatory markers: Elevated inflammatory markers like C-reactive protein are associated with both diabetes complications and ED.

Oxidative damage: Free radicals generated by high blood sugar damage the cellular machinery necessary for healthy erectile function.

Endothelial dysfunction: Inflammation and oxidative stress damage the endothelium, making blood vessels less responsive to arousal signals.

7. Structural Changes in Penile Tissue

Over time, chronic hyperglycemia can cause structural changes in erectile tissue:

Fibrosis: Scar tissue formation in the corpora cavernosa reduces the expandability of erectile chambers.

Smooth muscle changes: The smooth muscle cells that control blood flow may be replaced by fibrous tissue.

Venous leak: Damage to the mechanism that traps blood in the penis during erections can cause venous leak, where blood drains out too quickly to maintain rigidity.

Case Example: Thomas, Age 62

Thomas had well-controlled Type 1 diabetes for 35 years when he began experiencing ED. Unlike men with poor glucose control, Thomas had maintained an A1C below 7.0% for most of his diabetes duration.

"I was frustrated because I thought good control would prevent complications," Thomas explains. "My doctor explained that even with good control, long duration of diabetes can lead to some tissue changes."

Evaluation showed that Thomas had developed some degree of venous leak—blood was draining from his penis too quickly during erections. This is sometimes seen in men with long-standing diabetes, even when well-controlled.

Thomas's treatment included a combination of PDE5 inhibitors and constriction rings, which helped slow the drainage of blood during erections. He also began using a vacuum erection device on occasion.

"I had to adjust my expectations," Thomas says. "Perfect erections might not be realistic after 35 years of diabetes, but satisfying sex definitely is."

The Good News: What's Reversible

Understanding these mechanisms isn't meant to discourage you—it's meant to show you that there are multiple points where intervention can make a difference. Many of the factors that contribute to diabetes-related ED are modifiable.

Blood Sugar Control

Improving glucose control can help prevent further vascular and nerve damage and may even reverse some early changes. Studies show that men who achieve and maintain good glucose control have better sexual function outcomes.

Cardiovascular Health

Exercise, proper nutrition, and cardiovascular medications can improve blood flow throughout the body, including to the penis.

Weight Management

Weight loss improves insulin sensitivity, reduces inflammation, and can increase testosterone levels naturally.

Psychological Factors

Counseling, stress management, and treatment of depression can remove psychological barriers to sexual function.

Medication Optimization

Working with healthcare providers to minimize medications that interfere with sexual function while maintaining good diabetes control.

Hormone Optimization

Testosterone replacement therapy, when appropriate, can improve both libido and erectile function in men with low testosterone levels.

Early Intervention Benefits

The earlier you address diabetes-related ED, the better your outcomes are likely to be. Early intervention can:

- Prevent progression of vascular and nerve damage
- Maintain confidence and relationship satisfaction
- Identify and address other health issues
- Establish effective treatment approaches before problems become severe

Success Rate Statistics

The success rates for treating diabetes-related ED depend on several factors, including the severity of diabetes, the presence of other health conditions, and the specific treatments used:

- Lifestyle modifications alone: 30-40% improvement in mild to moderate ED
- PDE5 inhibitors: 60-70% success rate in men with diabetes (compared to 80% in men without diabetes)
- Combination approaches: 80-90% of men can achieve satisfactory sexual function with appropriate combination therapy
- Injection therapy: 85-90% success rate when properly used
- Penile implants: 90-95% satisfaction rates

Working With Your Body, Not Against It

The key to successful treatment of diabetes-related ED is understanding that you're not trying to override your diabetes—you're trying to optimize your health within the context of having diabetes.

This means:

- Accepting that treatment may be ongoing rather than a one-time fix
- Understanding that good diabetes management is foundational to sexual health
- Being willing to try different approaches to find what works best for you
- Recognizing that satisfying sexual function doesn't require perfect erections

Practical Tools

Visual Flowchart of Erection Process

1. Sexual stimulus (psychological or physical)
2. Brain processes arousal signals
3. Nerve signals travel to penis
4. Blood vessels in penis dilate
5. Blood flows into erectile chambers
6. Veins compress to trap blood
7. Erection achieved and maintained

Diabetes Disruption Points:

- High blood sugar → damaged blood vessels → reduced blood flow
- High blood sugar → nerve damage → impaired signal transmission
- Insulin resistance → low testosterone → reduced libido and erectile function
- Chronic stress → elevated cortisol → interference with arousal pathways

Personal Risk Factor Assessment

Rate your risk factors (1 = no concern, 5 = major concern):

- Blood sugar control (A1C level): ____
- Duration of diabetes: ____

- Blood pressure control: ___
- Cholesterol levels: ___
- Weight management: ___
- Stress levels: ___
- Medication side effects: ___
- Depression or anxiety: ___
- Smoking or alcohol use: ___
- Exercise level: ___

"Understanding My ED" Worksheet

1. How long have you had diabetes? ___
2. What's your most recent A1C? ___
3. How long have you noticed changes in sexual function? ___
4. Are the changes gradual or sudden? ___
5. Do you have other diabetes complications (neuropathy, retinopathy, nephropathy)? ___
6. What medications are you taking? ___
7. Have you had testosterone levels checked? ___
8. Are you experiencing stress, anxiety, or depression? ___

Understanding how diabetes affects your sexual function gives you a roadmap for treatment. Instead of seeing ED as a mysterious or insurmountable problem, you can now recognize it as a predictable consequence of diabetes that can be addressed systematically.

The next chapter will guide you through the process of getting a proper diagnosis and evaluation. Armed with this understanding of how diabetes affects sexual function, you'll be better prepared to work with your healthcare providers to identify the specific factors contributing to your ED and develop an effective treatment plan.

Remember that knowledge is power. The more you understand about your condition, the better equipped you are to make informed decisions about treatment and to achieve the best possible outcomes.

Key Takeaways:

- Normal erections require coordination of vascular, neurological, hormonal, and psychological systems
- Diabetes affects all systems necessary for healthy erectile function through seven distinct pathways
- Vascular damage from high blood sugar is the most common cause of diabetes-related ED
- Many factors contributing to ED are modifiable through proper treatment
- Early intervention leads to better outcomes than waiting for problems to worsen
- Success rates for treatment are high when appropriate approaches are used
- Understanding the mechanisms helps you work with healthcare providers more effectively
- Good diabetes management is foundational to sexual health improvement

Chapter 3: Getting the Right Diagnosis

Walking into a healthcare provider's office to discuss erectile dysfunction ranks among the most difficult conversations many men will ever have. The embarrassment, shame, and vulnerability can feel overwhelming. Yet this conversation represents the crucial first step toward reclaiming your sexual health and, often, your overall well-being.

The diagnostic process for diabetes-related ED isn't just about confirming that you have a problem—it's about understanding the specific factors contributing to your situation so that treatment can be targeted and effective. A thorough evaluation can reveal not just sexual health issues, but other complications of diabetes that need attention, medication side effects that can be addressed, and psychological factors that impact treatment success.

Before Your Appointment

Preparation for your healthcare visit begins weeks before you walk through the door. The more information you can provide your healthcare team, the more accurate your diagnosis will be and the more effective your treatment plan can become.

Medical History Preparation Checklist

Start by gathering information about your diabetes history:

- Date of diabetes diagnosis
- Type of diabetes (Type 1, Type 2, or other)
- Most recent A1C values (ideally the last 2-3 results)
- History of diabetes complications (retinopathy, neuropathy, nephropathy)
- Current diabetes medications and dosages
- Blood pressure and cholesterol readings
- History of diabetic ketoacidosis or severe hypoglycemia

Document your sexual health history:

- When did you first notice changes in sexual function?
- Were the changes gradual or sudden?
- How often do you have morning erections?
- Do you experience adequate libido (sexual desire)?
- Can you achieve erections with masturbation?
- How firm are your erections on a scale of 1-10?
- How long do erections last?
- Do you experience premature ejaculation or delayed ejaculation?

Medication List Template

Create a comprehensive list of all medications, including:

Prescription medications: Include diabetes medications, blood pressure medications, cholesterol medications, antidepressants, and any other prescription drugs.

Over-the-counter medications: Include vitamins, supplements, pain relievers, and herbal remedies.

Dosage and frequency: Note how much you take and how often.

Duration of use: How long you've been taking each medication.

Side effects experienced: Any side effects you've noticed, particularly related to sexual function.

Partner Involvement Decisions

Consider whether and how to involve your partner in the diagnostic process:

Benefits of partner involvement:

- Partners can provide additional information about changes they've observed
- Shared understanding of the medical nature of the problem

- Joint participation in treatment decisions
- Reduced relationship stress and blame

Potential concerns:

- Privacy and confidentiality issues
- Embarrassment about discussing intimate details
- Different comfort levels with medical discussions
- Scheduling conflicts

Case Example: William, Age 51

William, a 51-year-old engineer with Type 2 diabetes for seven years, spent three months preparing for his appointment with a urologist. "I kept putting off the appointment because I didn't know what to say or what information they'd need," he recalls.

His preparation included tracking his sexual function in a diary for two weeks, gathering five years of lab results from his endocrinologist, and researching potential medication interactions. "I made a spreadsheet of all my medications and when I started each one," William explains. "I realized that my ED had gotten worse around the time I started taking a beta-blocker for blood pressure."

During his appointment, William's thorough preparation allowed the urologist to quickly identify that his beta-blocker was likely contributing to his ED, in addition to diabetes-related vascular changes. "The doctor was impressed with my preparation and said it saved us at least two appointments because we had all the information needed to start treatment immediately."

Essential Tests and What They Mean

A thorough evaluation for diabetes-related ED involves multiple types of testing. Understanding what each test measures and why it's important helps you participate actively in your care and understand your results.

Blood Work

Hemoglobin A1C: This test measures your average blood sugar control over the past 2-3 months. For men with diabetes-related ED, the A1C provides crucial information about the likelihood that vascular damage is contributing to sexual dysfunction.

- A1C less than 7.0%: Good control, less likely that current high blood sugar is actively worsening ED
- A1C 7.0-8.0%: Moderate control, some ongoing vascular damage likely
- A1C greater than 8.0%: Poor control, active vascular damage occurring

Testosterone levels: Both total and free testosterone should be measured, preferably in the morning when levels are highest. Low testosterone contributes to both decreased libido and erectile dysfunction.

- Total testosterone below 300 ng/dL: Likely contributing to sexual dysfunction
- Total testosterone 300-400 ng/dL: May be contributing, especially if symptoms are present
- Total testosterone above 400 ng/dL: Less likely to be a primary factor

Lipid panel: Cholesterol and triglyceride levels affect vascular health and erectile function.

- LDL cholesterol above 100 mg/dL: May contribute to vascular ED
- HDL cholesterol below 40 mg/dL: Increases vascular risk
- Triglycerides above 150 mg/dL: Associated with insulin resistance and ED

Thyroid function: Both hyperthyroidism and hypothyroidism can affect sexual function.

Kidney function: Advanced diabetic kidney disease can affect hormone levels and medication choices.

Prostate-specific antigen (PSA): Important baseline measurement, especially if testosterone replacement is being considered.

Vascular Assessments

Penile Doppler ultrasound: This test measures blood flow into and out of the penis. It's the gold standard for diagnosing vascular causes of ED.

The test involves injecting a medication (usually alprostadil) directly into the penis to stimulate an erection, then using ultrasound to measure blood flow. While this sounds uncomfortable, most men tolerate it well, and the information gained is invaluable.

Normal results:

- Peak systolic velocity: 35-40 cm/sec or higher
- End diastolic velocity: Less than 5 cm/sec
- Resistive index: 0.8 or higher

Abnormal results indicating vascular ED:

- Peak systolic velocity: Less than 25 cm/sec (arterial insufficiency)
- End diastolic velocity: Greater than 5 cm/sec (venous leak)

Ankle-brachial index (ABI): This simple test compares blood pressure in your arms and legs to detect peripheral artery disease, which often correlates with penile artery disease.

Neurological Evaluations

Biothesiometry: This test measures vibratory sensation in the penis and can detect early nerve damage.

Nocturnal penile tumescence testing: This test monitors erections during sleep. Men typically have 3-5 erections during REM sleep, regardless of dream content. Absence of nocturnal erections suggests physical rather than psychological causes of ED.

Psychological Screening Tools

Beck Depression Inventory: This standardized questionnaire screens for depression, which affects up to 25% of men with diabetes.

International Index of Erectile Function (IIEF): This validated questionnaire assesses all aspects of sexual function, including erectile function, libido, and satisfaction.

Anxiety screening: Various questionnaires can identify anxiety disorders that may contribute to sexual dysfunction.

Case Example: Antonio, Age 44

Antonio, a 44-year-old restaurant manager with Type 2 diabetes for five years, underwent comprehensive testing after experiencing gradual worsening of ED over 18 months.

His blood work revealed:

- A1C: 8.4% (indicating poor diabetes control)
- Total testosterone: 225 ng/dL (low)
- LDL cholesterol: 145 mg/dL (elevated)
- HDL cholesterol: 32 mg/dL (low)

Penile Doppler ultrasound showed:

- Peak systolic velocity: 22 cm/sec (indicating arterial insufficiency)
- Normal venous function

Psychological screening revealed mild depression (Beck Depression Inventory score of 18).

"The testing showed me that my ED wasn't just one thing," Antonio explains. "My diabetes control was poor, my testosterone was low, my cholesterol was high, and I was dealing with some depression. It was actually reassuring to know that there were specific things we could fix."

Antonio's treatment plan addressed multiple factors: improved diabetes medications to lower his A1C, testosterone replacement therapy, a statin for cholesterol, counseling for depression, and PDE5 inhibitors for the vascular component of his ED.

"Six months later, my A1C was 7.1%, my testosterone was normal, my cholesterol was controlled, and my sexual function was dramatically better," Antonio reports. "The comprehensive testing let us treat everything at once instead of guessing."

Building Your Healthcare Team

Diabetes-related ED often requires a team approach. While your primary care provider can handle many aspects of diagnosis and treatment, certain situations benefit from specialist involvement.

Primary Care Coordination

Your primary care provider (family medicine, internal medicine, or endocrinology) should be the quarterback of your care. They can:

- Optimize diabetes management
- Screen for and treat depression
- Manage blood pressure and cholesterol
- Coordinate care between specialists
- Monitor for medication interactions
- Provide ongoing support and follow-up

When to See Specialists

Urologist: Consider urology referral for:

- Complex diagnostic testing (Doppler ultrasound)
- Failure of first-line treatments
- Consideration of injection therapy
- Penile implant evaluation
- Complex medical history

Endocrinologist: Consider endocrinology referral for:

- Difficult-to-control diabetes
- Hormone abnormalities
- Complex diabetes medication regimens
- Multiple diabetes complications

Mental Health Professionals: Consider referral for:

- Significant anxiety or depression
- Relationship counseling
- Sex therapy
- Substance abuse issues

Telemedicine Options and Benefits

Telemedicine has revolutionized the treatment of ED, particularly for men who find in-person visits embarrassing or difficult to schedule.

Benefits of telemedicine for ED:

- Increased privacy and comfort
- Better access to specialists
- More convenient follow-up appointments
- Often lower costs than in-person visits
- Ability to involve partners more easily

Limitations of telemedicine:

- Physical examination limitations
- Inability to perform certain tests
- Potential prescription limitations in some states
- Technology barriers for some patients

Case Example: Robert, Age 67

Robert, a 67-year-old retired mechanic living in rural Montana, had limited access to specialists for his diabetes-related ED. His nearest urologist was 200 miles away, and scheduling appointments required taking time off work for his wife to drive him.

"The telemedicine option changed everything for us," Robert explains. "I could talk to a specialist from home, my wife could be involved in the conversation, and we didn't have to lose a whole day traveling."

Robert's telemedicine consultation included:

- Detailed medical history review
- Discussion of his symptoms and concerns
- Review of recent lab work ordered by his primary care provider
- Development of a treatment plan
- Prescription for ED medication
- Scheduled follow-up appointments

"The doctor explained everything clearly, answered all our questions, and I felt just as comfortable as I would have in person," Robert says. "Actually, I felt more comfortable because I was in my own home."

The telemedicine approach allowed Robert to try multiple treatment approaches with regular follow-up, ultimately finding success with a combination of lifestyle changes and oral medication.

Practical Tools

Doctor Visit Preparation Template

Before your appointment, prepare answers to these questions:

1. What specific sexual function changes have you noticed?
2. When did these changes begin?

3. How have the changes progressed over time?
4. What makes symptoms better or worse?
5. How is your overall relationship satisfaction?
6. What are your goals for treatment?
7. What concerns do you have about treatment?
8. Are there any treatments you definitely want to avoid?

Test Results Tracking Log

Create a simple table to track your results over time:

Date | Test | Result | Normal Range | Notes

Example:

- 3/15/2024 | A1C | 8.2% | <7.0% | Need better control
- 3/15/2024 | Total T | 285 ng/dL | 300-1000 | Low, discuss replacement
- 3/15/2024 | PSA | 1.2 ng/mL | <4.0 | Normal baseline

Questions to Ask Your Provider Checklist

About your diagnosis:

- What specific factors are contributing to my ED?
- How does my diabetes control affect my sexual function?
- Are any of my medications contributing to the problem?
- What other health issues should we address?

About treatment options:

- What treatments do you recommend for my situation?
- What are the success rates for these treatments?
- What are the potential side effects?
- How quickly should I expect to see improvement?
- What if the first treatment doesn't work?

About follow-up:

- When should I follow up?
- What warning signs should I watch for?
- Who should I contact with questions or concerns?
- How will we monitor progress?

Healthcare Team Contact Organizer

Keep contact information organized:

Primary Care Provider:

- Name: _____
- Phone: _____
- Email/Portal: _____
- Best times to call: _____

Specialists:

- Urologist: _____
- Endocrinologist: _____
- Mental Health: _____

Emergency Contacts:

- After-hours number: _____
- Urgent care location: _____
- Hospital preference: _____

Setting Expectations for Your Visit

Understanding what to expect during your appointment can reduce anxiety and help you make the most of your time with your healthcare provider.

Initial Consultation

Your first visit will likely include:

- Detailed medical and sexual history
- Physical examination (including genital examination)
- Discussion of treatment goals and preferences
- Ordering of appropriate blood work
- Initial treatment recommendations
- Scheduling of follow-up appointments

The physical examination, while potentially embarrassing, is usually brief and professional. Your provider is looking for signs of hormone deficiency, circulation problems, nerve damage, or anatomical abnormalities.

Follow-up Visits

Subsequent visits typically focus on:

- Review of test results
- Assessment of treatment response
- Adjustment of medications or treatment approaches
- Monitoring for side effects
- Discussion of additional treatment options

Advocating for Comprehensive Care

Don't be afraid to advocate for thorough evaluation and appropriate treatment. Remember that:

- ED is a medical condition that deserves proper attention
- Comprehensive testing leads to better treatment outcomes
- You have the right to ask questions and understand your care
- Second opinions are appropriate if you're not satisfied with your initial evaluation
- Treatment should address all contributing factors, not just symptoms

The Road to Recovery Starts Here

Getting the right diagnosis is the foundation of successful treatment for diabetes-related ED. A thorough evaluation identifies all the factors contributing to your sexual dysfunction and allows for targeted, effective treatment.

The process may seem overwhelming, but remember that thousands of men go through this evaluation every year with positive outcomes. Your healthcare providers are there to help, not to judge, and modern medicine offers more effective treatments for diabetes-related ED than ever before.

The next chapter will help you take the information from your diagnostic evaluation and use it to create a personalized treatment plan that matches your specific situation, preferences, and goals.

Key Takeaways:

- Proper preparation before your appointment improves diagnostic accuracy and treatment outcomes
- Comprehensive testing identifies all factors contributing to your ED, not just diabetes
- Blood work, vascular testing, and psychological screening all play important roles in diagnosis
- A healthcare team approach often provides better results than single-provider care
- Telemedicine offers convenient, private access to specialist care for many men
- Advocacy for thorough evaluation is appropriate and leads to better outcomes
- The diagnostic process is the foundation for successful treatment of diabetes-related ED

Chapter 4: Creating Your Personalized Treatment Plan

The test results are in, the diagnosis is clear, and now comes the moment that matters most: deciding how to move forward. Creating an effective treatment plan for diabetes-related erectile dysfunction isn't a one-size-fits-all process. Your plan must consider your specific medical situation, personal preferences, relationship factors, financial circumstances, and lifestyle requirements.

This chapter will guide you through the decision-making process systematically, helping you understand all available options and how to match treatments to your unique circumstances. The goal isn't to find the "perfect" treatment—it's to find the approach that works best for your life and gives you the best chance of achieving satisfying sexual function.

Treatment Options Overview

Modern medicine offers a spectrum of treatments for diabetes-related ED, ranging from simple lifestyle modifications to sophisticated surgical interventions. Understanding the full menu of options helps you make informed decisions and sets realistic expectations.

First-Line Treatments

Lifestyle modifications: Diet, exercise, weight loss, smoking cessation, and improved diabetes control form the foundation of all ED treatment. These approaches address root causes rather than just symptoms.

- Effectiveness: 30-40% improvement in mild to moderate ED
- Timeline: 3-6 months for full benefit
- Cost: Variable, often cost-saving long-term
- Side effects: None when properly implemented

Oral medications (PDE5 inhibitors): Sildenafil (Viagra), tadalafil (Cialis), vardenafil (Levitra), and avanafil (Stendra) are the first-line medical treatments for ED.

- Effectiveness: 60-70% success rate in men with diabetes
- Timeline: Work within 30-60 minutes
- Cost: $10-50 per dose for brand names, $1-5 per dose for generics
- Side effects: Headache, flushing, nasal congestion, rare vision changes

Second-Line Treatments

Vacuum erection devices (VEDs): Mechanical devices that use suction to draw blood into the penis and constriction rings to maintain erections.

- Effectiveness: 70-80% of men can achieve erections adequate for intercourse
- Timeline: Immediate effect
- Cost: $150-500 for quality devices
- Side effects: Bruising, numbness, unnatural feeling

Injection therapy: Direct injection of medications into the penis to produce erections independent of nerve function or blood flow problems.

- Effectiveness: 85-90% success rate when properly used
- Timeline: Erection within 5-15 minutes
- Cost: $15-30 per injection
- Side effects: Pain, priapism (rare), scarring (rare)

Intraurethral therapy: Suppositories placed in the urethra that are absorbed locally to produce erections.

- Effectiveness: 40-60% success rate
- Timeline: Erection within 10-30 minutes
- Cost: $25-40 per dose
- Side effects: Urethral burning, dizziness

Third-Line Treatments

Penile implants: Surgical placement of devices inside the penis that allow men to achieve erections mechanically.

- Effectiveness: 90-95% satisfaction rates
- Timeline: 6-8 weeks recovery, then immediate function
- Cost: $15,000-25,000 (often covered by insurance)
- Side effects: Surgical risks, potential for mechanical failure

Emerging Treatments

Low-intensity shockwave therapy: Sound waves applied to penile tissue to stimulate blood vessel growth and nerve regeneration.

- Effectiveness: 60-70% improvement in mild to moderate ED
- Timeline: Series of treatments over 6-12 weeks
- Cost: $3,000-6,000 for complete series
- Side effects: Minimal, mild discomfort during treatment

Platelet-rich plasma (PRP): Injection of concentrated platelets from the patient's own blood to promote tissue healing and regeneration.

- Effectiveness: Limited data, 50-60% improvement reported
- Timeline: Multiple treatments over several months
- Cost: $1,500-3,000 per treatment
- Side effects: Minimal, injection site discomfort

Effectiveness Rates by Diabetes Severity

The success of ED treatments varies significantly based on the severity and duration of diabetes, overall health status, and the presence of diabetes complications.

Well-Controlled Diabetes (A1C < 7.0%)

Men with well-controlled diabetes generally have better treatment outcomes across all modalities:

- PDE5 inhibitors: 70-80% success rate
- Injection therapy: 90-95% success rate
- Vacuum devices: 80-85% success rate
- Lifestyle modifications: 40-50% improvement

Moderately Controlled Diabetes (A1C 7.0-8.5%)

Moderate glucose control shows intermediate success rates:

- PDE5 inhibitors: 60-70% success rate
- Injection therapy: 85-90% success rate
- Vacuum devices: 75-80% success rate
- Lifestyle modifications: 30-40% improvement

Poorly Controlled Diabetes (A1C > 8.5%)

Poor diabetes control significantly reduces treatment effectiveness:

- PDE5 inhibitors: 45-60% success rate
- Injection therapy: 80-85% success rate
- Vacuum devices: 70-75% success rate
- Lifestyle modifications: 20-30% improvement (but glucose control improvement can dramatically increase success rates)

Case Example: Frank, Age 56

Frank, a 56-year-old construction supervisor with Type 2 diabetes for 12 years, came to treatment with an A1C of 9.8% and severe ED. His initial trial of sildenafil 100mg showed minimal improvement.

"I was ready to give up," Frank recalls. "The doctor said the pills would work for most men, but they barely helped me at all."

Rather than moving immediately to more invasive treatments, Frank's healthcare team focused first on diabetes control. Over four months, medication adjustments and lifestyle changes brought his A1C down to 7.6%.

"Once my blood sugar got better, we tried the pills again," Frank explains. "The difference was dramatic. The same dose that barely worked before was now giving me solid erections."

Frank's case illustrates how improved diabetes control can significantly enhance the effectiveness of ED treatments. His success with oral medication improved from about 20% to 80% simply by optimizing his glucose control first.

Cost Considerations with 2024-2025 Pricing

Understanding the financial aspects of ED treatment helps you make realistic decisions and plan for ongoing expenses.

Oral Medications (Monthly Costs)

Brand name PDE5 inhibitors:

- Viagra (sildenafil): $400-500 per month for 8 doses
- Cialis (tadalafil): $450-550 per month for daily dosing
- Levitra (vardenafil): $350-450 per month for 8 doses
- Stendra (avanafil): $400-500 per month for 8 doses

Generic PDE5 inhibitors:

- Generic sildenafil: $20-40 per month for 8 doses
- Generic tadalafil: $30-50 per month for daily dosing
- Generic vardenafil: $25-45 per month for 8 doses

Cost-saving strategies:

- Insurance coverage verification
- Manufacturer discount programs
- Online pharmacy options
- Pill splitting (when medically appropriate)
- Generic substitution

Injection Therapy (Per-Dose Costs)

Single-agent injections:

- Alprostadil (Caverject): $25-35 per dose
- Alprostadil (Edex): $25-35 per dose

Compounded multi-agent injections:

- Trimix (alprostadil/phentolamine/papaverine): $8-15 per dose
- Bimix (papaverine/phentolamine): $6-12 per dose
- Quadmix (adds atropine): $10-18 per dose

Device Costs (One-Time Purchases)

Vacuum erection devices:

- Basic manual pumps: $150-300
- Battery-operated pumps: $300-500
- Prescription devices: $400-600 (often insurance covered)

Constriction rings:

- Basic rings: $10-25 each
- Adjustable rings: $30-50 each
- Sets with multiple sizes: $50-100

Surgical Costs (One-Time Procedures)

Penile implants:

- Inflatable implants: $18,000-25,000
- Semi-rigid implants: $15,000-20,000
- Revision surgeries: $20,000-30,000

Insurance coverage: Medicare and most insurance plans cover penile implants when medical necessity is documented.

Case Example: George, Age 49

George, a 49-year-old small business owner without prescription drug coverage, faced significant financial challenges in treating his diabetes-related ED.

"The brand-name pills were $50 each, and I needed them twice a week," George explains. "That's $400 per month just for sex—more than my car payment."

George worked with his healthcare provider to find cost-effective solutions:

1. Generic sildenafil reduced his per-dose cost from $50 to $3
2. A manufacturer discount program provided additional savings
3. His provider prescribed 100mg tablets to split into 50mg doses, halving the cost
4. Quarterly visits instead of monthly visits reduced healthcare costs

"With these changes, my monthly cost went from $400 to about $40," George says. "That made treatment sustainable for my budget."

Decision-Making Framework

Choosing the right treatment approach requires systematic consideration of multiple factors. This framework helps organize your decision-making process.

Medical Factors

Severity of ED:

- Mild ED: Often responds well to lifestyle changes and oral medications
- Moderate ED: May require combination approaches or second-line treatments
- Severe ED: Often needs injection therapy or surgical options

Diabetes control status:

- Well-controlled: All treatment options likely to be effective
- Poorly controlled: Focus on glucose control first, then reassess options

Other health conditions:

- Heart disease: May limit some medication options
- Blood pressure medications: May interact with ED treatments
- Antidepressants: May reduce effectiveness of some treatments

Previous treatment history:

- Failed oral medications: Consider injection therapy or devices
- Needle phobia: Avoid injection therapy
- Previous pelvic surgery: May affect treatment options

Personal Preferences

Spontaneity vs. planning:

- High spontaneity preference: Daily tadalafil or injection therapy
- Comfort with planning: As-needed oral medications

Invasiveness tolerance:

- Non-invasive preference: Oral medications and lifestyle changes
- Comfort with procedures: Injection therapy or surgery

Partner involvement:

- Partner supportive: Any treatment option viable
- Partner squeamish: Avoid injection therapy or devices

Relationship Factors

Frequency of sexual activity:

- Infrequent (less than weekly): As-needed treatments
- Regular (weekly or more): Daily medications or long-acting options

Partner's preferences:

- Supports any effective treatment: All options open
- Prefers "natural" approaches: Lifestyle changes and oral medications
- Wants minimal interference: Long-acting or surgical options

Lifestyle Considerations

Travel requirements:

- Frequent travel: Oral medications or implants
- Minimal travel: Any option appropriate

Privacy concerns:

- High privacy needs: Oral medications or surgery
- Comfortable with visible devices: Vacuum devices acceptable

Time availability:

- Limited time: Quick-acting oral medications
- Flexible schedule: Devices or injection therapy

Case Example: Carl, Age 61

Carl, a 61-year-old retiree with Type 2 diabetes for 15 years, worked through the decision framework with his wife Janet to choose the best treatment approach.

Medical factors:

- Moderate to severe ED
- Well-controlled diabetes (A1C 7.2%)
- Taking blood pressure medication that contributed to ED
- Previous failure with sildenafil

Personal preferences:

- Wanted reliable, predictable results
- Comfortable with some invasiveness
- Janet supportive of any effective treatment

Relationship factors:

- Sexual activity 2-3 times per week
- 35-year marriage with open communication
- Both wanted to return to satisfying sexual relationship

Lifestyle considerations:

- Retired with flexible schedule
- Privacy at home
- Occasional travel to visit children

"We went through all the options systematically," Carl explains. "Janet and I talked about what mattered most to us—reliability and getting back to a normal sex life."

After considering all factors, Carl chose injection therapy with trimix. "The thought of injections was scary at first, but the 90% success rate and reliable results made it worth trying," he says.

Six months later, Carl and Janet report excellent results. "The injections work every time, and after the first few uses, they became routine," Carl notes. "It's given us our sex life back."

Setting Realistic Expectations

One of the most important aspects of treatment planning is establishing realistic expectations. Unrealistic expectations lead to disappointment and treatment abandonment, while appropriate expectations lead to satisfaction and adherence.

Timeline for Improvement by Treatment Type

Lifestyle modifications:

- Initial improvements: 4-6 weeks
- Significant improvements: 3-6 months
- Maximum benefit: 6-12 months

Oral medications:

- Immediate trial: Same day
- Optimal dosing: 2-4 weeks of trials
- Maximum effectiveness: 4-8 weeks

Injection therapy:

- Learning proper technique: 2-4 weeks
- Optimal dosing: 4-6 weeks
- Consistent results: 6-8 weeks

Vacuum devices:

- Learning technique: 2-3 weeks
- Comfortable use: 4-6 weeks
- Optimal results: 6-8 weeks

Surgical options:

- Recovery from surgery: 6-8 weeks
- Full function: 8-12 weeks
- Complete adaptation: 3-6 months

Combination Therapy Benefits

Many men achieve optimal results by combining multiple treatment approaches:

Lifestyle + oral medications: Improved effectiveness and potentially lower medication doses needed.

Oral medications + vacuum devices: Better rigidity and longer-lasting erections.

Injection therapy + constriction rings: More reliable results and potentially lower injection doses.

Any treatment + counseling: Better overall satisfaction and relationship quality.

When to Adjust Your Plan

Treatment plans should be dynamic, not static. Consider adjustments when:

- No improvement after appropriate trial period
- Partial improvement that's not satisfactory
- Side effects that affect quality of life
- Changes in health status or medications
- Changes in relationship or lifestyle factors
- New treatment options become available

Practical Tools

Treatment Decision Tree

Start with these questions to guide your initial treatment choice:

1. Is your diabetes well-controlled (A1C < 7.5%)?
   - No: Focus on glucose control first
   - Yes: Proceed to question 2
2. Have you tried lifestyle modifications for at least 3 months?
   - No: Start with lifestyle changes

- o   Yes: Proceed to question 3
3. Are you comfortable taking oral medications?
    - o   Yes: Trial PDE5 inhibitors
    - o   No: Consider injection therapy or devices
4. Did oral medications provide satisfactory results?
    - o   Yes: Continue with optimization
    - o   No: Consider second-line treatments
5. Are you comfortable with injection therapy?
    - o   Yes: Trial injection therapy
    - o   No: Consider vacuum devices or surgery

Cost-Benefit Calculator

For each treatment option, calculate:

Monthly cost:

- Medication costs
- Device costs (amortized)
- Healthcare visit costs

Effectiveness rating (1-10 scale based on your specific situation)

Convenience rating (1-10 scale based on your preferences)

Overall value = (Effectiveness × Convenience) ÷ Cost

SMART Goals Worksheet for Sexual Health

Create Specific, Measurable, Achievable, Relevant, Time-bound goals:

Example:

- Specific: Achieve erections firm enough for penetration
- Measurable: Success rate of 70% or higher
- Achievable: Using appropriate medical treatment
- Relevant: Important for relationship satisfaction

- Time-bound: Within 3 months of starting treatment

Your goals:

1. _____
2. _____
3. _____

Treatment Tracking Log

Track your progress systematically:

Date | Treatment | Dose/Setting | Effectiveness (1-10) | Side Effects | Notes

This tracking helps identify patterns and optimize your treatment approach.

The Journey Ahead

Creating your personalized treatment plan is just the beginning of your journey back to satisfying sexual function. The plan you develop today may evolve as you gain experience with different treatments, as your health changes, or as new options become available.

Remember that successful treatment often requires patience, persistence, and sometimes multiple attempts to find the optimal approach. The men who achieve the best outcomes are those who stay engaged in the process, communicate openly with their healthcare providers and partners, and remain flexible in their approach.

The next section of this book will walk you through the specific treatments in detail, starting with lifestyle modifications that form the foundation of all successful ED treatment. Armed with your personalized plan, you'll be ready to implement these treatments systematically and effectively.

Key Takeaways:

- Treatment success depends on matching the right approach to your specific situation
- Diabetes control significantly affects the success of all ED treatments
- Cost considerations are important for sustainable treatment plans
- Realistic expectations lead to better treatment satisfaction
- Combination approaches often provide better results than single treatments
- Treatment plans should be flexible and adjust based on results and changing circumstances
- Systematic decision-making frameworks help choose optimal treatments for your situation

Chapter 5: Lifestyle Medicine

Most men seeking treatment for diabetes-related erectile dysfunction want a pill or procedure that will instantly solve their problem. This desire for a quick fix is understandable—ED affects not just sexual function but self-esteem, relationships, and overall quality of life. However, the most successful treatment approaches for diabetes-related ED begin with lifestyle modifications that address the root causes of the problem rather than just masking symptoms.

Lifestyle medicine isn't about becoming a perfect health specimen or making dramatic life changes overnight. It's about making strategic, sustainable modifications that improve blood flow, reduce inflammation, optimize hormone levels, and enhance overall vascular health. These changes don't just improve erectile function—they often improve diabetes control, reduce cardiovascular risk, and increase energy and well-being.

The Mediterranean Approach to Sexual Health

The Mediterranean diet has garnered significant attention in recent years, not just for heart health and diabetes management, but specifically for its benefits on erectile function. Research shows that men who follow a Mediterranean-style eating pattern have significantly lower rates of ED and better response to ED treatments when needed.

Why the Mediterranean Diet Works for ED

The Mediterranean approach addresses multiple pathways that contribute to diabetes-related ED:

Improved endothelial function: Foods rich in antioxidants and healthy fats help restore the function of blood vessel linings, improving blood flow throughout the body, including to the penis.

Reduced inflammation: The anti-inflammatory properties of Mediterranean foods help reduce the chronic inflammation that damages blood vessels and interferes with erectile function.

Better insulin sensitivity: This eating pattern improves how your body responds to insulin, leading to better glucose control and reduced diabetes-related vascular damage.

Increased nitric oxide production: Many Mediterranean foods contain compounds that support nitric oxide production, the key chemical messenger for penile blood vessel dilation.

Specific Foods That Improve Blood Flow

Fatty fish (salmon, mackerel, sardines, anchovies): Rich in omega-3 fatty acids that improve blood vessel function and reduce inflammation. Aim for 2-3 servings per week.

Leafy greens (spinach, arugula, kale): High in nitrates that convert to nitric oxide in the body. Include 1-2 servings daily.

Nuts and seeds (walnuts, almonds, pistachios, flaxseeds): Provide healthy fats, protein, and compounds that support vascular health. A handful (1 ounce) daily is optimal.

Berries (blueberries, strawberries, raspberries): Packed with antioxidants called anthocyanins that improve blood flow and reduce inflammation.

Dark chocolate (70% cacao or higher): Contains flavonoids that improve blood vessel function. Limit to 1-2 ounces daily.

Olive oil (extra virgin): Rich in monounsaturated fats and antioxidants that support cardiovascular health. Use as your primary cooking fat.

Tomatoes (especially cooked): High in lycopene, an antioxidant that improves blood flow and may specifically benefit erectile function.

Garlic and onions: Contain compounds that improve circulation and may have direct benefits for sexual function.

Foods to Limit or Avoid

Processed meats: High in saturated fat and sodium, which can worsen vascular function.

Refined sugars and simple carbohydrates: Cause blood sugar spikes that damage blood vessels over time.

Trans fats: Found in some processed foods, these fats directly harm blood vessel function.

Excessive alcohol: While moderate red wine consumption may have benefits, excessive alcohol impairs sexual function.

High-sodium foods: Can worsen blood pressure and vascular function.

Case Example: Miguel, Age 52

Miguel, a 52-year-old accountant with Type 2 diabetes for eight years, had been struggling with gradually worsening ED for two years. His typical diet consisted of fast food lunches, processed dinners, and minimal fruits or vegetables.

"I knew my diet wasn't great, but I didn't think it was connected to my sex life," Miguel admits. "I thought ED was just something that happened with diabetes."

Working with a registered dietitian, Miguel gradually transitioned to a Mediterranean-style eating pattern over three months:

Breakfast: Changed from sugary cereal to Greek yogurt with berries and nuts *Lunch*: Replaced fast food with salads containing olive oil, nuts, and grilled fish or chicken *Dinner*: Shifted from processed meals to home-cooked dishes featuring lean proteins, vegetables, and whole grains *Snacks*: Swapped chips and cookies for nuts, fruits, and vegetables

"The changes were gradual, so they didn't feel overwhelming," Miguel explains. "After about six weeks, I noticed I had more energy. After three months, my morning erections were coming back."

Miguel's three-month results:

- A1C decreased from 8.1% to 7.3%
- Weight loss of 18 pounds
- Blood pressure improved from 145/92 to 132/84
- Significant improvement in erectile function (IIEF score increased from 12 to 19)
- Improved energy and mood

"The diet changes didn't just help with ED—I felt better overall," Miguel reflects. "My diabetes control improved, my energy was better, and my wife said I seemed happier."

Exercise as Medicine

Regular physical activity is one of the most powerful interventions for diabetes-related ED, yet it's often overlooked in favor of medications or devices. Exercise addresses ED through multiple mechanisms: improving cardiovascular fitness, enhancing blood flow, reducing inflammation, improving insulin sensitivity, boosting testosterone levels naturally, and reducing stress and anxiety.

The 45-60 Minute Daily Protocol

Research shows that men who exercise for 45-60 minutes daily have significantly better erectile function than sedentary men. This doesn't mean you need to become a marathon runner or spend hours in the gym—it means incorporating regular, moderate-intensity activity into your daily routine.

Aerobic exercise (30-40 minutes daily):

- Brisk walking at a pace where you can talk but feel slightly breathless
- Swimming, cycling, or elliptical machine workouts
- Dancing, hiking, or recreational sports
- Target heart rate: 50-70% of maximum (220 minus your age)

Resistance training (20-30 minutes, 3 times per week):

- Focus on major muscle groups (legs, back, chest, shoulders, arms)
- Use weights, resistance bands, or bodyweight exercises
- Aim for 8-12 repetitions that challenge your muscles
- Progressive overload: gradually increase resistance over time

Flexibility and stress reduction (10-15 minutes daily):

- Yoga, stretching, or tai chi
- Deep breathing exercises
- Progressive muscle relaxation

Starting Safely with Diabetes

Exercise with diabetes requires attention to blood sugar management and potential complications:

Get medical clearance: Especially important if you have diabetes complications like retinopathy, neuropathy, or cardiovascular disease.

Start gradually: Begin with 10-15 minutes of activity and increase by 5 minutes per week until you reach your target.

Monitor blood glucose: Check before, during (for longer sessions), and after exercise.

Stay hydrated: Diabetes increases dehydration risk during exercise.

Foot care: Inspect feet daily and wear proper footwear to prevent injuries.

Timing considerations: Exercise after meals can help control blood sugar spikes.

Tracking Blood Sugar During Exercise

Safe exercise with diabetes requires understanding how physical activity affects your blood glucose:

Pre-exercise glucose levels:

- Less than 100 mg/dL: Eat 15-30g carbohydrates before exercising
- 100-180 mg/dL: Safe to exercise
- 180-250 mg/dL: Exercise with caution, monitor closely
- Above 250 mg/dL: Check for ketones; avoid exercise if ketones are present

During exercise:

- Monitor for signs of hypoglycemia (shaking, sweating, confusion)
- For sessions longer than 60 minutes, check glucose every 30 minutes
- Have fast-acting carbohydrates available

Post-exercise:

- Blood sugar can continue to drop for 4-24 hours after exercise
- Monitor more frequently, especially overnight
- May need to reduce insulin doses on exercise days

Case Example: Robert, Age 58

Robert, a 58-year-old office manager with Type 1 diabetes for 25 years, had been sedentary for most of his adult life. When ED began affecting his marriage, his endocrinologist recommended exercise as part of his treatment plan.

"I hadn't exercised regularly since high school," Robert admits. "The idea of starting at my age with diabetes seemed overwhelming and risky."

Robert started with a conservative approach:

Week 1-2: 10-minute walks after dinner, monitoring blood sugar before and after *Week 3-4*: Increased to 15-minute walks, added light stretching *Week 5-8*: Built up to 30-minute walks, added resistance bands twice weekly *Week 9-12*: Progressed to 45-minute combination of walking and basic strength exercises

"The key was starting slowly and tracking everything," Robert explains. "I kept a log of my blood sugar, exercise time, and how I felt. It helped me learn how my body responded to different activities."

Robert's exercise log showed patterns that helped optimize his routine:

- Walking after meals helped control post-meal blood sugar spikes
- Morning exercise required a small snack to prevent hypoglycemia
- His insulin needs decreased by about 15% on exercise days
- His overnight blood sugars were more stable on days he exercised

After six months of consistent exercise:

- A1C improved from 7.8% to 7.1%
- Lost 22 pounds and gained noticeable muscle tone
- Blood pressure decreased from 142/88 to 128/82
- Reported significant improvement in energy and mood
- IIEF score improved from 14 to 21, indicating moderate improvement in erectile function
- Testosterone levels increased from 285 ng/dL to 380 ng/dL

"The exercise didn't just help with ED—it improved everything," Robert reflects. "My diabetes control got better, I felt stronger and more confident, and my overall health improved dramatically."

Weight Loss That Lasts

Obesity significantly worsens diabetes-related ED through multiple mechanisms: increased insulin resistance, reduced testosterone levels, impaired blood flow, increased inflammation, and psychological factors affecting self-esteem and sexual confidence.

The 5-15% Solution

You don't need to achieve "ideal" body weight to see significant improvements in sexual function. Research consistently shows that losing just 5-15% of body weight can lead to meaningful improvements in erectile function, diabetes control, and overall health.

For a 220-pound man:

- 5% weight loss = 11 pounds (down to 209 pounds)
- 10% weight loss = 22 pounds (down to 198 pounds)
- 15% weight loss = 33 pounds (down to 187 pounds)

Sustainable Weight Loss Strategies

Calorie balance: Create a moderate calorie deficit of 500-750 calories per day through a combination of reduced intake and increased activity. This leads to 1-2 pounds of weight loss per week.

Portion control: Use smaller plates, measure portions initially to calibrate your perception, and focus on eating slowly to recognize satiety signals.

Meal timing: Regular meal times help regulate blood sugar and may improve insulin sensitivity. Avoid skipping meals, which can lead to overeating later.

Macronutrient balance: Aim for 45-65% of calories from carbohydrates (focusing on complex carbs), 20-35% from fat (emphasizing healthy fats), and 10-35% from protein.

Hydration: Often, thirst is mistaken for hunger. Drink water before meals and throughout the day.

GLP-1 Medications and Sexual Function

A new class of diabetes medications called GLP-1 receptor agonists (semaglutide/Ozempic, liraglutide/Victoza, dulaglutide/Trulicity) has shown remarkable effectiveness for weight loss in addition to diabetes control. Emerging research suggests these medications may have direct benefits for sexual function:

Weight loss effects: Significant weight loss improves insulin sensitivity, reduces inflammation, and can increase testosterone levels naturally.

Cardiovascular benefits: Improved heart health translates to better blood flow throughout the body, including to the penis.

Potential direct effects: Some research suggests GLP-1 medications may have direct effects on blood vessel function and nitric oxide production.

Blood sugar control: Better glucose control reduces ongoing vascular damage.

Case Example: Dennis, Age 45

Dennis, a 45-year-old restaurant owner with Type 2 diabetes for six years, weighed 285 pounds when he began experiencing ED. His A1C was 9.2%, and he felt trapped in a cycle of poor eating habits driven by long work hours and stress.

"I was surrounded by food all day at work, stressed about the business, and eating terribly," Dennis explains. "I knew I needed to lose weight, but I'd tried diets before and always gained it back."

Dennis's healthcare team prescribed semaglutide (Ozempic) as part of a comprehensive approach that included:

Dietary changes:

- Worked with a dietitian to develop realistic meal plans for his work schedule
- Pre-planned healthy options at his restaurant
- Focused on high-protein, high-fiber foods that promoted satiety

Exercise integration:

- Started with 20-minute walks before opening the restaurant
- Used a fitness tracker to monitor daily steps
- Added resistance training twice weekly at a nearby gym

Medication management:

- Semaglutide helped reduce appetite and cravings
- Metformin dosage was optimized
- Blood pressure medication was adjusted as weight decreased

Dennis's 12-month results were remarkable:

- Weight loss of 67 pounds (from 285 to 218 pounds)
- A1C improvement from 9.2% to 6.8%
- Blood pressure normalization (discontinued blood pressure medication)
- Testosterone levels increased from 235 ng/dL to 425 ng/dL
- Significant improvement in erectile function (IIEF score from 8 to 22)
- Reported dramatic improvements in energy, mood, and self-confidence

"The weight loss changed everything," Dennis says. "Not just the ED, but how I felt about myself, my energy level, even how I ran my business. My wife says I'm like a different person."

Sleep, Stress, and Sexual Health

The connection between sleep, stress, and sexual function is often overlooked but critically important for men with diabetes-related ED.

The Sleep Apnea Connection

Sleep apnea affects up to 80% of men with Type 2 diabetes and significantly worsens both diabetes control and erectile function:

Oxygen deprivation: Repeated episodes of low oxygen during sleep damage blood vessels throughout the body.

Hormone disruption: Sleep apnea reduces testosterone production and increases stress hormones.

Inflammation: Poor sleep quality increases inflammatory markers that worsen vascular function.

Blood sugar control: Sleep apnea worsens insulin resistance and makes diabetes harder to control.

Signs of sleep apnea include loud snoring, witnessed breathing pauses during sleep, morning headaches, excessive daytime sleepiness, and difficulty concentrating.

Stress Hormone Impacts

Chronic stress releases cortisol and adrenaline, which directly interfere with sexual function:

Cortisol effects: Suppresses testosterone production, increases blood sugar, and impairs immune function.

Adrenaline effects: Constricts blood vessels, making erections more difficult to achieve and maintain.

Psychological effects: Chronic stress increases anxiety and depression, which further worsen sexual function.

Practical Stress Reduction Techniques

Deep breathing exercises:

- Practice 4-7-8 breathing: inhale for 4 counts, hold for 7, exhale for 8
- Use throughout the day, especially before sexual activity

Progressive muscle relaxation:

- Systematically tense and relax muscle groups from head to toe
- Helps identify and release physical tension

Mindfulness meditation:

- Even 10 minutes daily can reduce stress hormones
- Apps like Headspace or Calm provide guided sessions

Regular sleep schedule:

- Go to bed and wake up at consistent times
- Aim for 7-9 hours of sleep nightly
- Create a relaxing bedtime routine

Time management:

- Prioritize important tasks
- Delegate when possible
- Say no to non-essential commitments

Case Example: Paul, Age 41

Paul, a 41-year-old paramedic with Type 2 diabetes for four years, worked rotating shifts that severely disrupted his sleep patterns. He began experiencing ED during a particularly stressful period at work.

"I was working overtime constantly, sleeping at weird hours, and drinking too much coffee to stay alert," Paul explains. "My blood sugars were all over the place, and my sex life disappeared."

Paul's sleep study revealed severe sleep apnea with an apnea-hypopnea index (AHI) of 42 events per hour (normal is less than 5). His healthcare team addressed multiple factors:

Sleep apnea treatment:

- CPAP therapy normalized his breathing during sleep
- Lost 25 pounds, which reduced apnea severity
- Improved sleep quality dramatically

Stress management:

- Learned relaxation techniques for use before and after shifts
- Started regular exercise routine compatible with shift work
- Worked with scheduling supervisor to reduce mandatory overtime

Diabetes optimization:

- Continuous glucose monitor helped track patterns during different shifts
- Medication timing was adjusted for shift work
- A1C improved from 8.6% to 7.4%

Paul's results after six months:

- Sleep quality improved dramatically with CPAP therapy
- Energy levels increased significantly
- Blood sugar control improved markedly
- Testosterone levels increased from 275 ng/dL to 395 ng/dL
- IIEF score improved from 11 to 19
- Relationship stress decreased, overall mood improved

"Getting my sleep fixed was like getting my life back," Paul reflects. "I had no idea how much the sleep apnea was affecting everything— my diabetes, my energy, my sex life, even my mood."

Practical Tools

4-Week Lifestyle Change Starter Kit

Week 1: Foundation

- Track current eating patterns and blood sugar responses
- Add 15-minute walk after dinner daily
- Establish consistent sleep schedule
- Begin stress reduction practice (5 minutes daily)

Week 2: Building

- Introduce one Mediterranean diet principle (e.g., olive oil as primary fat)
- Increase exercise to 20-25 minutes daily
- Add one serving of vegetables to each meal
- Continue stress reduction practice

Week 3: Expanding

- Add resistance training twice weekly
- Increase vegetable and fruit intake
- Reduce processed food consumption by 50%
- Increase stress reduction to 10 minutes daily

Week 4: Optimizing

- Exercise 30-40 minutes daily (mix of aerobic and resistance)
- Follow Mediterranean eating pattern 80% of the time
- Establish consistent meal timing
- Evaluate progress and plan next month

Blood Sugar and Exercise Tracking Template

Date | Pre-Exercise BG | Exercise Type | Duration | Post-Exercise BG | Notes

Example: 3/15/24 | 145 mg/dL | Brisk walk | 30 min | 115 mg/dL | Felt energized, no symptoms

Mediterranean Diet Shopping Lists

Proteins:

- Fatty fish (salmon, mackerel, sardines)
- Lean poultry
- Eggs
- Legumes (beans, lentils, chickpeas)
- Greek yogurt

Healthy Fats:

- Extra virgin olive oil
- Nuts (walnuts, almonds, pistachios)
- Seeds (flax, chia, hemp)
- Avocados
- Olives

Carbohydrates:

- Leafy greens (spinach, arugula, kale)
- Colorful vegetables (tomatoes, peppers, broccoli)
- Berries (blueberries, strawberries, raspberries)
- Whole grains (quinoa, brown rice, oats)

Flavor enhancers:

- Garlic and onions
- Fresh herbs (basil, oregano, parsley)
- Lemon and lime
- Dark chocolate (70% cacao or higher)

Progress Photo Guidelines

Take monthly progress photos to track changes:

- Same time of day (preferably morning)
- Same lighting and location
- Same clothing or lack thereof
- Front, side, and back views
- Include face (captures overall health improvements)
- Take measurements (waist, chest, arms, thighs)

The Foundation for Everything Else

Lifestyle modifications form the foundation upon which all other ED treatments build. Men who implement these changes often find that medications work better, devices are more effective, and surgical outcomes are improved. More importantly, these changes address the root causes of diabetes-related ED rather than just treating symptoms.

The key to success with lifestyle medicine is understanding that small, consistent changes compound over time. You don't need to transform your entire life overnight. Start with one or two changes, master them, then gradually add others. The men who achieve lasting success are those who make sustainable changes they can maintain long-term.

Remember that lifestyle medicine isn't about perfection—it's about progress. Every healthy meal, every exercise session, every good night's sleep moves you closer to better sexual function and overall health. These changes take time to show their full effects, but they create lasting improvements that extend far beyond the bedroom.

Essential Insights:

- Lifestyle modifications address root causes of diabetes-related ED, not just symptoms
- The Mediterranean diet improves blood flow, reduces inflammation, and supports vascular health

- Exercise for 45-60 minutes daily significantly improves erectile function in men with diabetes
- Weight loss of just 5-15% can lead to meaningful improvements in sexual function
- Sleep quality and stress management are often overlooked but critical factors
- GLP-1 medications may provide benefits beyond glucose control and weight loss
- Small, consistent changes compound over time to create significant improvements
- Lifestyle changes enhance the effectiveness of other ED treatments

Chapter 6: Medications That Work

After implementing lifestyle changes and optimizing diabetes control, many men find they still need medical treatments to achieve satisfactory sexual function. This isn't a failure—it's a recognition that diabetes-related ED often requires a combination of approaches for optimal results. Modern medicine offers several effective medication options, each with distinct advantages, limitations, and ideal use cases.

Understanding how these medications work, their effectiveness in men with diabetes, and how to use them properly can mean the difference between treatment success and disappointment. This chapter will guide you through the medication options available, help you understand what to expect, and provide practical guidance for getting the best results from whichever approach you choose.

Oral Medications (PDE5 Inhibitors)

Phosphodiesterase type 5 (PDE5) inhibitors revolutionized ED treatment when sildenafil (Viagra) was first introduced in 1998. These medications work by blocking an enzyme that breaks down cyclic GMP, the chemical messenger responsible for penile smooth muscle relaxation and blood vessel dilation during erections.

How PDE5 Inhibitors Work

During sexual arousal, nerve signals trigger the release of nitric oxide in penile tissue. Nitric oxide activates an enzyme called guanylate cyclase, which produces cyclic GMP. Cyclic GMP causes smooth muscle relaxation and blood vessel dilation, allowing blood to flow into the penis and create an erection.

The enzyme PDE5 naturally breaks down cyclic GMP, ending the erection. PDE5 inhibitors block this enzyme, allowing cyclic GMP levels to remain elevated longer, resulting in firmer, longer-lasting erections.

Why They Work Less Well with Diabetes

Men with diabetes often have reduced effectiveness with PDE5 inhibitors due to several factors:

Reduced nitric oxide production: High blood sugar damages the cells that produce nitric oxide, reducing the initial signal that PDE5 inhibitors amplify.

Vascular damage: Damaged blood vessels may not respond normally to cyclic GMP signals, even when levels are elevated.

Nerve damage: Diabetic neuropathy can interfere with the nerve signals that initiate the nitric oxide cascade.

Advanced atherosclerosis: Severe blood vessel disease may prevent adequate blood flow despite medication.

Despite these challenges, PDE5 inhibitors remain effective for 60-70% of men with diabetes, compared to 80-85% effectiveness in men without diabetes.

Sildenafil (Viagra) - The Pioneer

Sildenafil was the first PDE5 inhibitor and remains one of the most widely used:

Dosing: Available in 25mg, 50mg, and 100mg tablets. Most men start with 50mg and adjust based on effectiveness and side effects.

Timing: Take 30-60 minutes before sexual activity. Peak effectiveness occurs 1-2 hours after taking the medication.

Duration: Effects last 4-6 hours, though this doesn't mean you'll have an erection for this entire time—you need sexual stimulation for the medication to work.

Food interactions: High-fat meals can delay absorption and reduce effectiveness. Take on an empty stomach or with a light meal for best results.

Cost: Generic sildenafil costs $1-3 per tablet, while brand-name Viagra costs $50-70 per tablet.

Tadalafil (Cialis) - The Weekend Pill

Tadalafil offers unique advantages due to its longer duration of action:

Dosing: Available in 2.5mg, 5mg, 10mg, and 20mg tablets. Can be used as-needed (10-20mg) or daily (2.5-5mg).

Timing: As-needed dosing works within 30 minutes and lasts up to 36 hours. Daily dosing provides continuous readiness.

Duration: Up to 36 hours for as-needed dosing, making it ideal for men who prefer spontaneity or have sexual activity on multiple days.

Food interactions: Can be taken with or without food—meals don't significantly affect absorption.

Additional benefits: Also approved for benign prostatic hyperplasia (BPH), so may help with urinary symptoms in addition to ED.

Cost: Generic tadalafil costs $1-4 per tablet for as-needed use, $30-50 per month for daily dosing.

Vardenafil (Levitra) - The Rapid Response

Vardenafil offers some advantages in terms of onset and food interactions:

Dosing: Available in 5mg, 10mg, and 20mg tablets. Most men start with 10mg.

Timing: Works within 25-30 minutes, slightly faster than sildenafil.

Duration: Effects last 4-6 hours, similar to sildenafil.

Food interactions: Less affected by fatty meals than sildenafil, but still works best on an empty stomach.

Selectivity: More selective for PDE5 than sildenafil, potentially meaning fewer side effects.

Cost: Generic vardenafil costs $2-5 per tablet.

Avanafil (Stendra) - The Fast Track

Avanafil is the newest PDE5 inhibitor, designed for rapid onset:

Dosing: Available in 50mg, 100mg, and 200mg tablets.

Timing: Can work as quickly as 15 minutes after taking, making it the fastest-acting PDE5 inhibitor.

Duration: Effects last approximately 6 hours.

Food interactions: Minimal interaction with food or alcohol.

Side effects: May have fewer side effects due to greater selectivity for PDE5.

Cost: Currently only available as brand-name, costing $40-60 per tablet.

Case Example: Richard, Age 54

Richard, a 54-year-old sales manager with Type 2 diabetes for nine years, had tried sildenafil with limited success. His A1C was well-controlled at 7.1%, but he was experiencing moderate ED that interfered with his 28-year marriage.

"I tried Viagra first because it's what everyone knows about," Richard explains. "It worked sometimes, but not consistently enough to feel confident about planning intimate time with my wife."

Richard worked with his urologist to optimize his PDE5 inhibitor therapy:

Trial 1: Sildenafil 50mg - Worked about 60% of the time, with headaches as a side effect.

Trial 2: Increased sildenafil to 100mg - Better effectiveness (75%) but more severe headaches.

Trial 3: Switched to tadalafil 20mg as-needed - Good effectiveness (80%) with minimal side effects.

Trial 4: Changed to daily tadalafil 5mg - Consistent effectiveness (85%) and improved spontaneity.

"The daily Cialis was a game-changer," Richard says. "I didn't have to plan around taking a pill, and it worked reliably. The spontaneity really improved our relationship."

Richard's final regimen:

- Daily tadalafil 5mg taken every morning
- Excellent diabetes control maintained
- Consistent erectile function adequate for satisfying intercourse
- No significant side effects
- Improved relationship satisfaction and reduced performance anxiety

Daily vs. On-Demand Dosing

The choice between daily and as-needed dosing depends on several factors:

Daily Dosing Advantages:

- Provides continuous readiness for sexual activity
- Eliminates need to plan around medication timing
- May improve treatment effectiveness over time
- Reduces performance anxiety related to medication timing
- Potential cardiovascular benefits from continuous PDE5 inhibition

Daily Dosing Considerations:

- Higher monthly cost
- Continuous medication exposure
- May be prescribed primarily with tadalafil due to its safety profile

As-Needed Dosing Advantages:

- Lower cost (only pay when using)
- Avoid continuous medication exposure
- Can adjust dose based on specific situations
- Works with all PDE5 inhibitors

As-Needed Dosing Considerations:

- Requires planning around sexual activity
- May contribute to performance anxiety
- Less consistent blood levels of medication

Generic Cost-Saving Strategies

The availability of generic PDE5 inhibitors has dramatically reduced treatment costs:

Generic Availability:

- Sildenafil: Generic available since 2017
- Tadalafil: Generic available since 2018
- Vardenafil: Generic available since 2020
- Avanafil: Still brand-name only

Cost Reduction Strategies:

Insurance coverage verification: Check formulary coverage and prior authorization requirements.

Pill splitting: Higher-strength tablets often cost the same as lower-strength tablets. A 100mg sildenafil tablet split in half provides two 50mg doses at half the per-dose cost.

Online pharmacies: Legitimate online pharmacies often offer significant savings, especially for cash-paying customers.

Manufacturer programs: Most manufacturers offer discount programs for uninsured or underinsured patients.

Compounding pharmacies: Some compounding pharmacies offer lower-cost alternatives, though quality may vary.

International pharmacies: While potentially risky, some men use Canadian or other international pharmacies for cost savings.

The Game Changer: Eroxon Topical Gel

In 2023, the FDA approved the first over-the-counter topical treatment for ED: Eroxon gel. This represents a significant advancement in ED treatment, particularly for men who prefer non-oral options or have contraindications to PDE5 inhibitors.

How Eroxon Works

Eroxon uses a unique mechanism called "dynamic cooling" that doesn't rely on the nitric oxide pathway:

Physical stimulation: The gel creates a cooling sensation followed by warming as it's absorbed, stimulating nerve endings in the glans (head) of the penis.

Neurogenic response: This stimulation triggers reflexive dilation of penile blood vessels through nerve pathways rather than chemical pathways.

Rapid onset: Because it works through physical stimulation rather than systemic absorption, effects can begin within 5-10 minutes.

How to Use Eroxon

Application: Apply the entire contents of one tube to the glans of the penis and massage gently for 15 seconds.

Timing: Use immediately before sexual activity—no need to wait 30-60 minutes like oral medications.

Frequency: Can be used up to once daily.

Partner considerations: The gel may transfer to partners, though clinical trials showed no safety concerns.

Best Candidates for Eroxon

Men who cannot take PDE5 inhibitors: Those with heart conditions, taking nitrates, or experiencing intolerable side effects.

Men seeking rapid onset: Those who prefer not to plan sexual activity around medication timing.

Men with mild to moderate ED: Clinical trials showed best results in men with less severe ED.

Men preferring topical treatment: Those uncomfortable with oral medications or injections.

Real-World Effectiveness Data

Clinical trials of Eroxon showed:

- 65% of men achieved erections sufficient for intercourse
- Median time to erection: 10 minutes
- 80% of men found it easy to use
- No serious side effects reported
- Effectiveness maintained over 12 weeks of use

Case Example: Steven, Age 49

Steven, a 49-year-old firefighter with Type 2 diabetes for six years, couldn't take PDE5 inhibitors due to a heart condition that required nitrate medication for angina.

"I thought I was out of options," Steven explains. "My cardiologist said I couldn't take Viagra or Cialis because of my heart medication, and I wasn't ready for injections."

When Eroxon became available, Steven's urologist suggested trying it:

Initial trial: Used Eroxon according to instructions before sexual activity with his wife of 22 years.

Results: Achieved erections adequate for intercourse about 70% of the time, with onset typically within 8-12 minutes.

Side effects: Mild cooling sensation that both Steven and his wife found tolerable.

Cost: Approximately $25 per tube, with insurance not covering over-the-counter treatments.

"It's not perfect, but it gave me back an option when I thought I had none," Steven says. "The fact that it works so quickly is actually an advantage—we don't have to plan around medication timing."

Steven's experience highlights Eroxon's value for men who can't use other treatments and prefer the rapid onset it provides.

Injection Therapy

For men who don't respond adequately to oral medications or topical treatments, injection therapy offers an highly effective alternative. While the idea of injecting medication directly into the penis may seem daunting, most men find the process more tolerable than expected and appreciate the reliable results.

How Injection Therapy Works

Intracavernosal injections bypass the need for intact nerve pathways and adequate blood flow by directly introducing vasoactive medications into the erectile tissue. These medications cause immediate smooth muscle relaxation and blood vessel dilation, producing erections that are independent of arousal level or psychological factors.

Alprostadil (Caverject, Edex) - The Single Agent

Alprostadil is a synthetic version of prostaglandin E1, a naturally occurring compound that causes blood vessel dilation:

Mechanism: Directly stimulates adenylyl cyclase, increasing cyclic AMP levels and causing smooth muscle relaxation.

Effectiveness: 70-80% of men achieve erections adequate for intercourse.

Onset: Erections typically develop within 5-15 minutes.

Duration: Erections last 30-60 minutes regardless of orgasm.

Dosing: Starting doses range from 2.5-5 micrograms, adjusted based on response.

Cost: $25-35 per injection for brand-name products.

Trimix and Custom Compounds - The Power Combinations

Many men achieve better results with combination injections that include multiple medications:

Trimix composition:

- Alprostadil (prostaglandin E1): Causes blood vessel dilation
- Papaverine: Blocks calcium channels, promoting smooth muscle relaxation
- Phentolamine: Blocks alpha-adrenergic receptors, preventing vessel constriction

Advantages of combinations:

- Higher success rates (85-95%)
- Often lower doses of individual medications needed
- Reduced side effects from any single agent
- More consistent, predictable results

Bimix: Contains only papaverine and phentolamine, used for men who can't tolerate alprostadil.

Quadmix: Adds atropine to Trimix, which may improve effectiveness in some men.

Cost: $8-15 per injection from compounding pharmacies.

Injection Technique Mastery

Proper injection technique is crucial for safety and effectiveness:

Injection site: Into the corpus cavernosum (erectile chamber) on either side of the penis, avoiding the urethra and major blood vessels.

Needle size: Typically 29-30 gauge needles, which are very thin and cause minimal discomfort.

Injection depth: Approximately 1/2 to 3/4 inch, depending on penis size.

Angle: Perpendicular to the penis shaft.

Rotation: Alternate injection sites to prevent scar tissue formation.

Sterile technique: Clean hands, sterile needles, and alcohol wipes to prevent infection.

Managing the Fear Factor

The psychological barrier to injection therapy is often the biggest obstacle:

Education: Understanding that the injection is virtually painless helps reduce anxiety.

Gradual exposure: Starting with very low doses and gradually increasing builds confidence.

Partner support: Having a supportive partner who understands the medical necessity helps.

Professional guidance: Learning proper technique from healthcare providers ensures safety and effectiveness.

Success reinforcement: Experiencing reliable results helps overcome initial hesitation.

Case Example: David, Age 61

David, a 61-year-old retired teacher with Type 1 diabetes for 32 years, had developed significant diabetic complications including neuropathy and vascular disease. Oral medications provided minimal benefit, and his ED was severely affecting his 35-year marriage.

"I was terrified of the injections," David admits. "The thought of sticking a needle in my penis seemed impossible. But my ED was so bad that we barely had any intimacy left."

David's injection therapy journey:

Initial consultation: His urologist explained the procedure and safety profile in detail.

First injection: Performed in the doctor's office with alprostadil 5 micrograms. Achieved firm erection lasting 45 minutes with minimal discomfort.

Home training: Nurse practitioner taught David and his wife proper injection technique.

Dose optimization: Switched to Trimix and found optimal dose of 0.15ml that produced reliable erections lasting 30-45 minutes.

Long-term use: After two years of injection therapy, David reports 95% success rate with no significant side effects.

"The injections completely changed our lives," David explains. "After the first few times, they became routine. The reliability is amazing— we know it will work every time, which eliminated all the performance anxiety."

David's wife, Margaret, adds: "I was worried about the injections too, but seeing how much it helped David's confidence and our relationship made it worthwhile. It gave us back our intimacy."

Intraurethral Options

Intraurethral therapy offers a needle-free alternative for men who want medication-based treatment but can't tolerate injections.

MUSE (Medicated Urethral System for Erection)

MUSE delivers alprostadil through a small suppository inserted into the urethra:

Mechanism: Alprostadil is absorbed through urethral tissue and diffuses into the erectile chambers.

Application: Small suppository is inserted about 1 inch into the urethra using a plastic applicator.

Effectiveness: 40-60% of men achieve erections adequate for intercourse.

Side effects: Urethral burning, dizziness (due to blood pressure effects), and minor bleeding are possible.

Partner effects: Female partners may experience vaginal burning if medication transfers during intercourse.

When to Consider Intraurethral Therapy

Needle phobia: Men who cannot overcome fear of injections.

Injection contraindications: Men with bleeding disorders or taking blood thinners.

Moderate ED: Best results in men with less severe erectile dysfunction.

Trial option: As a step between oral medications and injection therapy.

Case Example: Mark, Age 55

Mark, a 55-year-old nurse with Type 2 diabetes for eight years, had moderate ED that didn't respond well to oral medications. His medical background made him knowledgeable about injection therapy, but he had a lifelong needle phobia.

"I knew injections would probably work better, but I just couldn't get past the needle fear," Mark explains. "As a nurse, I've given thousands of injections, but the thought of injecting my penis was overwhelming."

Mark tried MUSE with mixed results:

- Achieved adequate erections about 50% of the time
- Experienced mild urethral burning initially
- Found the application process straightforward
- Appreciated the needle-free approach

After six months with MUSE, Mark eventually overcame his needle phobia and switched to injection therapy for more reliable results. "MUSE was a good bridge that let me experience medication-based treatment without needles," he reflects. "It built my confidence to eventually try injections."

Combination Approaches

Many men achieve optimal results by combining different treatment modalities:

Oral Medications + Lifestyle Optimization

- Improved diabetes control enhances PDE5 inhibitor effectiveness
- Weight loss and exercise can restore natural erectile function
- Combination often allows lower medication doses

PDE5 Inhibitors + Vacuum Devices

- Medication improves blood flow while device provides mechanical assistance
- Particularly effective for men with moderate vascular damage

Injection Therapy + Constriction Rings

- Rings help maintain erections achieved through injections
- May allow lower injection doses

- Useful for men with venous leak

Practical Tools

Medication Comparison Chart with 2025 Costs

Sildenafil (Generic):

- Onset: 30-60 minutes
- Duration: 4-6 hours
- Cost: $1-3 per dose
- Food effects: Significant

Tadalafil (Generic):

- Onset: 30 minutes
- Duration: Up to 36 hours
- Cost: $1-4 per dose (as-needed), $30-50/month (daily)
- Food effects: Minimal

Vardenafil (Generic):

- Onset: 25-30 minutes
- Duration: 4-6 hours
- Cost: $2-5 per dose
- Food effects: Moderate

Eroxon Gel:

- Onset: 5-10 minutes
- Duration: Variable
- Cost: $25 per application
- Food effects: None

Trimix Injection:

- Onset: 5-15 minutes
- Duration: 30-60 minutes

- Cost: $8-15 per dose
- Food effects: None

Side Effect Management Guide

Headaches: Start with lower doses, stay hydrated, consider switching medications.

Flushing: Common and usually mild, typically improves with continued use.

Nasal congestion: Try nasal decongestants, consider switching to different PDE5 inhibitor.

Visual changes: Rare but serious—seek immediate medical attention.

Priapism (erection lasting >4 hours): Medical emergency—seek immediate treatment.

Injection Anxiety Reduction Protocol

1. *Education phase*: Learn about safety and effectiveness
2. *Visualization*: Practice mental rehearsal of injection process
3. *Partner involvement*: Include supportive partner in learning process
4. *Professional demonstration*: Watch healthcare provider perform first injection
5. *Supervised practice*: Perform injection under professional supervision
6. *Home practice*: Start with lowest effective dose
7. *Gradual independence*: Build confidence through successful experiences

Insurance Coverage Worksheet

Check formulary coverage for:

- Brand-name PDE5 inhibitors

- Generic PDE5 inhibitors
- Prior authorization requirements
- Quantity limits per month
- Injection therapy coverage
- Vacuum device coverage

Document:

- Copay amounts for each option
- Annual deductible status
- Prior authorization approval process
- Appeals process if denied

Moving Beyond Pills

While oral medications remain the first-line treatment for most men with diabetes-related ED, they're just one tool in a comprehensive treatment toolkit. The key to successful treatment often lies in finding the right combination of approaches that work for your specific situation.

Understanding your medication options empowers you to work effectively with your healthcare providers to find the approach that gives you the best results with the fewest side effects. Whether that's optimizing your response to oral medications, exploring topical options like Eroxon, or considering injection therapy, each option offers genuine hope for restored sexual function.

The next chapter will explore device-based treatments that can work independently or in combination with medications to provide mechanical solutions for erectile dysfunction. These options are particularly valuable for men who don't respond adequately to medications alone or who prefer non-pharmaceutical approaches.

Key Treatment Insights:

- PDE5 inhibitors work for 60-70% of men with diabetes, though effectiveness may be reduced compared to men without diabetes
- Generic versions of most PDE5 inhibitors have dramatically reduced treatment costs
- Daily dosing with tadalafil offers advantages in spontaneity and consistent effectiveness
- Eroxon gel provides a rapid-acting, over-the-counter option for men who can't use oral medications
- Injection therapy offers 85-95% success rates but requires overcoming psychological barriers
- Combination approaches often provide better results than single treatments
- Cost considerations and insurance coverage significantly impact treatment accessibility
- Proper technique and realistic expectations are crucial for treatment success

Chapter 7: Devices and Mechanical Solutions

When medications alone don't provide satisfactory results, or when men prefer non-pharmaceutical approaches, mechanical devices offer effective alternatives for achieving and maintaining erections. These solutions work through physical mechanisms rather than chemical pathways, making them particularly valuable for men with advanced diabetes complications that affect nerve function or blood flow.

Device-based treatments range from external vacuum systems that can be used as needed, to internal penile implants that provide permanent solutions. While the idea of mechanical assistance may initially seem unnatural or concerning, millions of men worldwide have found these devices restore satisfying sexual function and dramatically improve quality of life.

Vacuum Erection Devices (VEDs)

Vacuum erection devices, also known as penis pumps, represent one of the most straightforward and effective non-pharmaceutical treatments for ED. These devices work by creating a vacuum around the penis, drawing blood into the erectile chambers, then using a constriction ring to maintain the erection.

How Vacuum Devices Work

The VED system consists of three main components:

Cylinder: A clear plastic tube that fits over the penis, creating an airtight seal against the body.

Pump mechanism: Either manual (hand-operated) or battery-powered, this creates the vacuum that draws blood into the penis.

Constriction rings: Elastic or adjustable rings that slide from the base of the cylinder onto the base of the penis to maintain the erection.

The process works by creating negative pressure around the penis, which causes blood to flow into the erectile chambers (corpora cavernosa). Once adequate firmness is achieved, the constriction ring is moved to the base of the penis to trap blood and maintain the erection. The cylinder is then removed, leaving the ring in place during sexual activity.

Choosing FDA-Approved Devices

The FDA regulates vacuum devices as medical devices, and choosing an approved device ensures safety and quality standards:

Prescription devices: Available through healthcare providers, often covered by insurance, and include professional guidance on proper use.

Over-the-counter devices: Available without prescription but vary widely in quality and safety features.

Quality indicators: Look for devices with pressure gauges to prevent over-pumping, comfortable seals, and durable construction.

Reputable manufacturers: Companies like Coloplast (Pos-T-Vac), Boston Scientific (VED), and Timm Medical have established track records for quality and safety.

Proper Technique for Best Results

Successful use of vacuum devices requires proper technique and patience:

Preparation:

- Trim pubic hair around the base of the penis for better seal
- Apply water-based lubricant to the penis and cylinder opening
- Ensure the device is clean and the battery (if applicable) is charged

Application:

- Place the cylinder over the penis, pressing firmly against the body to create a seal
- Begin pumping slowly and steadily—rapid pumping can cause injury
- Monitor pressure and stop if pain or discomfort occurs

Vacuum creation:

- Pump until the penis becomes firm enough for intercourse
- This typically takes 2-5 minutes of gradual pumping
- The penis may appear darker or feel cooler than normal—this is expected

Ring placement:

- Quickly move the constriction ring from the cylinder base to the penis base
- Ensure the ring is positioned at the very base of the penis
- Remove the cylinder carefully

Duration limits:

- Keep the ring in place for no more than 30 minutes
- Remove immediately if pain, numbness, or color changes occur
- Wait at least 60 minutes between uses

Partner Involvement Strategies

Including your partner in VED use can improve both effectiveness and relationship satisfaction:

Education: Help your partner understand how the device works and why it's necessary.

Participation: Some couples find that having the partner operate the device makes it feel more natural and intimate.

Timing: Incorporate device use into foreplay rather than treating it as a medical procedure.

Communication: Discuss expectations and concerns openly to reduce anxiety for both partners.

Patience: Allow time to become comfortable with the device— proficiency improves with practice.

Case Example: Harold, Age 67

Harold, a 67-year-old retired electrician with Type 2 diabetes for 18 years, had developed significant vascular disease that made oral medications ineffective. His wife of 42 years, Dorothy, was supportive but initially skeptical about vacuum devices.

"I wasn't sure about using a machine for something that used to be so natural," Harold admits. "Dorothy was worried it would be awkward or painful."

Harold's VED journey:

Initial trial: His urologist provided an in-office demonstration with a prescription device.

Learning curve: The first few attempts at home were frustrating, with difficulty achieving adequate vacuum and proper ring placement.

Partner involvement: Dorothy began helping with the device operation, which reduced Harold's anxiety and improved their intimacy.

Technique refinement: Over several weeks, they developed a routine that incorporated the device into their foreplay.

Long-term success: After six months, Harold achieved satisfactory erections for intercourse 80% of the time.

"It took some getting used to, but it gave us back our sex life," Harold explains. "Dorothy says she doesn't even notice the ring during intercourse, and the erections are firm enough for both of us to enjoy."

Dorothy adds: "I was worried it would feel mechanical or unromantic, but helping Harold with it actually brought us closer together. We had to communicate more about what worked and what didn't."

Effectiveness and Expectations

VED effectiveness varies based on several factors:

Overall success rates: 70-80% of men can achieve erections adequate for intercourse.

Diabetes-specific outcomes: Men with diabetes may have slightly lower success rates due to vascular complications.

Continuation rates: About 65% of men continue using VEDs long-term, with discontinuation often due to inconvenience rather than ineffectiveness.

Partner satisfaction: Studies show that partners are generally satisfied with VED use when properly educated about the process.

Expected characteristics of VED-assisted erections:

- Firmness adequate for penetration but may feel different than natural erections
- Reduced sensation at the base of the penis due to the constriction ring
- Slightly cooler temperature and darker color due to altered blood flow
- Ability to maintain erection after orgasm (until ring is removed)

- Some men experience reduced ejaculation force due to ring pressure

Penile Implants - The Permanent Solution

For men who don't achieve satisfactory results with other treatments, or who prefer a permanent solution, penile implants represent the most definitive treatment for ED. These surgically placed devices allow men to achieve erections mechanically, independent of blood flow, nerve function, or psychological factors.

Three Types Explained Simply

Inflatable three-piece implants: The most sophisticated option, consisting of two inflatable cylinders in the penis, a fluid reservoir in the abdomen, and a pump in the scrotum. When activated, fluid moves from the reservoir to the cylinders, creating an erection that closely mimics natural firmness and appearance.

Inflatable two-piece implants: Similar to three-piece systems but combine the pump and reservoir in the scrotum. Slightly less natural-feeling than three-piece systems but easier to implant.

Semi-rigid (malleable) implants: Consist of bendable rods placed in the penis that can be positioned up for intercourse or down for concealment. Always firm but can be bent into position as needed.

What Surgery Really Involves

Penile implant surgery is typically performed as an outpatient procedure under general or spinal anesthesia:

Surgical approach: The surgeon makes a small incision either at the base of the penis or in the lower abdomen.

Preparation: The erectile chambers (corpora cavernosa) are dilated to accommodate the implant cylinders.

Implant placement: Cylinders are inserted into the erectile chambers, and additional components (reservoir, pump) are positioned as appropriate for the implant type.

Closure: Incisions are closed with absorbable sutures, and the patient is monitored during recovery.

Duration: The procedure typically takes 1-2 hours, depending on the complexity and surgeon experience.

Recovery timeline:

- *Hospital stay*: Usually outpatient or overnight observation
- *Pain management*: Moderate pain for 3-5 days, manageable with prescription medications
- *Activity restrictions*: No heavy lifting or strenuous activity for 4-6 weeks
- *Return to work*: 1-2 weeks for desk jobs, longer for physical labor
- *Sexual activity*: 6-8 weeks after surgery, once healing is complete
- *Full function*: 8-12 weeks for complete adaptation to the device

98.7% Medicare Coverage Facts

Penile implants have excellent insurance coverage when medical necessity is documented:

Medicare coverage: Medicare covers penile implants when ED is documented and other treatments have failed or are contraindicated.

Private insurance: Most private insurance plans cover implants with similar criteria to Medicare.

Documentation requirements: Medical records must show trial and failure of other treatments (medications, devices) or contraindications to other treatments.

Prior authorization: Most insurers require prior authorization, but approval rates are high when criteria are met.

Cost coverage: Insurance typically covers 80-90% of costs after deductibles are met.

70-90% Satisfaction Rates Explained

Penile implant satisfaction rates are among the highest of any medical procedure:

Patient satisfaction factors:

- Reliable, on-demand erections
- Natural appearance when not inflated (for inflatable types)
- Preservation of orgasm and ejaculation
- Improved sexual confidence
- Freedom from medication dependence

Partner satisfaction factors:

- Predictable sexual function
- Natural feel during intercourse
- Improved relationship dynamics
- Reduced performance anxiety for both partners

Factors affecting satisfaction:

- Realistic pre-surgical expectations
- Adequate post-operative counseling
- Proper device function
- Absence of complications

Case Example: Frank, Age 59

Frank, a 59-year-old mechanic with Type 1 diabetes for 28 years, had tried multiple treatments for his severe ED without success. Oral medications provided minimal benefit, injection therapy worked inconsistently, and vacuum devices were cumbersome for his active lifestyle.

"I was tired of dealing with medications and devices that sometimes worked and sometimes didn't," Frank explains. "My wife and I wanted reliability—something that would work every time without planning around pills or injections."

Frank's implant journey:

Decision process: After discussing options with his urologist, Frank chose a three-piece inflatable implant for the most natural feel.

Surgery: Outpatient procedure with no complications. Frank went home the same day.

Recovery: Experienced moderate pain for four days, managed with prescription medications. Returned to light duty work after two weeks.

Activation: At six weeks post-surgery, Frank learned to operate the device and had his first successful intercourse.

Long-term results: Two years later, Frank reports 100% success rate with no mechanical problems.

"The implant completely changed our lives," Frank says. "It works every single time, feels natural, and my wife can't tell the difference during intercourse. We have our spontaneity back."

Frank's wife, Linda, adds: "I was nervous about Frank having surgery, but the results have been amazing. He's more confident, we're more intimate, and there's no worry about whether treatments will work."

Comparing Implant Types

Three-Piece Inflatable Implants: *Advantages*: Most natural feel, best concealment when deflated, highest patient satisfaction

Disadvantages: Most complex surgery, highest cost, potential for mechanical failure *Best for*: Men seeking most natural function and appearance

Two-Piece Inflatable Implants: *Advantages*: Simpler than three-piece, good concealment, reliable function *Disadvantages*: Less natural feel than three-piece, limited reservoir volume *Best for*: Men who want inflatable function with simpler surgery

Semi-Rigid Implants: *Advantages*: Simplest surgery, lowest cost, highest reliability, easy to use *Disadvantages*: Always firm, more difficult to conceal, less natural feel *Best for*: Men with limited dexterity, those prioritizing simplicity and reliability

Constriction Rings and Combination Approaches

Constriction rings can be used alone or in combination with other treatments to enhance effectiveness:

Standalone Use:

- Effective for men with mild venous leak
- Helps maintain naturally occurring erections
- Can be used with or without medications

Combination with Vacuum Devices:

- Standard component of VED systems
- Essential for maintaining vacuum-assisted erections

Combination with Medications:

- Can enhance effectiveness of PDE5 inhibitors
- May allow lower medication doses
- Useful for men with partial response to medications

Combination with Injection Therapy:

- Can extend duration of injection-induced erections
- May allow lower injection doses
- Helps men with rapid detumescence

Safe Usage Guidelines:

- Never wear for more than 30 minutes
- Remove immediately if pain or numbness occurs
- Choose appropriate size (snug but not painful)
- Avoid metal rings that can't be cut off if stuck
- Clean thoroughly between uses

When Rings Help Most:

- Men with venous leak (blood draining too quickly from penis)
- Those seeking to extend duration of erections
- Men wanting to enhance effectiveness of other treatments
- Those with mild ED who can achieve but not maintain erections

Practical Tools

Device Comparison Matrix

Vacuum Erection Device:

- Effectiveness: 70-80%
- Invasiveness: None (external use)
- Cost: $200-500 one-time
- Spontaneity: Requires 5-10 minutes preparation
- Maintenance: Cleaning, occasional part replacement
- Insurance coverage: Often covered

Inflatable Penile Implant:

- Effectiveness: 90-95%
- Invasiveness: Surgical procedure
- Cost: $18,000-25,000 (usually covered by insurance)

- Spontaneity: Immediate activation
- Maintenance: Minimal, occasional mechanical issues
- Insurance coverage: Excellent

Semi-Rigid Implant:

- Effcctivcncss: 85-90%
- Invasiveness: Surgical procedure
- Cost: $15,000-20,000 (usually covered by insurance)
- Spontaneity: Always ready
- Maintenance: Minimal, highest reliability
- Insurance coverage: Excellent

Insurance Pre-Authorization Templates

Information needed for prior authorization:

- Complete medical history including diabetes duration and complications
- Documentation of previous ED treatments tried and their outcomes
- Current medications and contraindications to other treatments
- Impact of ED on quality of life and relationships
- Physician recommendation with medical rationale

Supporting documentation:

- Laboratory results (testosterone, A1C, lipids)
- Cardiac clearance if applicable
- Psychological evaluation if relevant
- Partner counseling documentation

Post-Surgery Recovery Timeline

Days 1-3:

- Pain management with prescribed medications
- Ice packs to reduce swelling
- Light activities only

- Monitor for signs of infection

Days 4-14:

- Gradual return to normal activities
- Avoid heavy lifting (>10 pounds)
- Keep incision sites clean and dry
- Follow-up appointment with surgeon

Weeks 3-6:

- Increasing activity as tolerated
- No sexual activity until cleared by surgeon
- Monitor device area for any concerns

Weeks 6-8:

- Device activation training
- First sexual activity
- Adjustment period for device use

Months 2-6:

- Complete adaptation to device
- Resolution of any minor issues
- Long-term satisfaction assessment

Partner Education Materials

What partners need to know about VEDs:

- How the device works and why it's necessary
- What to expect during use (appearance, feel, timing)
- How they can help with operation if desired
- Normal characteristics of device-assisted erections
- When to be concerned about problems

What partners need to know about implants:

- How the implant works and what surgery involves
- Recovery timeline and support needed
- What to expect when sexual activity resumes
- How the implant feels during intercourse
- Long-term reliability and satisfaction data

Making the Right Choice

Choosing between device options depends on multiple factors:

Consider VEDs if:

- You want a non-invasive, reversible option
- Cost is a primary concern
- You're comfortable with some preparation time
- Other treatments provide partial but insufficient benefit
- You want to try a mechanical approach before considering surgery

Consider implants if:

- You want maximum reliability and spontaneity
- Other treatments have failed or are contraindicated
- You're willing to undergo surgery for permanent solution
- Insurance coverage makes cost manageable
- You prioritize natural feel and appearance

Consider combination approaches if:

- Single treatments provide partial benefit
- You want to optimize effectiveness of existing treatments
- Cost-effectiveness is important
- You prefer gradual escalation of treatment intensity

The Technology Advantage

Device-based treatments offer unique advantages for men with diabetes-related ED:

Independence from vascular function: Mechanical solutions work regardless of blood vessel damage from diabetes.

Independence from nerve function: Devices don't require intact nerve pathways to function.

Reliability: Mechanical solutions provide consistent results not affected by blood sugar levels, stress, or medications.

Permanent solution potential: Implants provide long-term resolution without ongoing medication costs.

Combination benefits: Devices can enhance the effectiveness of other treatments.

Device-based treatments represent mature, well-established technologies with decades of successful use. While newer treatments continue to emerge, vacuum devices and penile implants remain gold standards for men who need reliable, effective solutions for diabetes-related ED.

The choice between devices and other treatments isn't about giving up or accepting defeat—it's about choosing the approach that best fits your lifestyle, preferences, and medical situation. Many men find that device-based treatments provide the reliability and spontaneity they need to maintain satisfying sexual relationships.

The next chapter will explore cutting-edge treatments that are emerging from research laboratories and clinical trials, offering hope for even more effective solutions in the future.

Essential Device Knowledge:

- Vacuum erection devices offer effective, non-invasive treatment with 70-80% success rates
- Proper technique and partner involvement significantly improve VED outcomes
- Penile implants provide the highest satisfaction rates (90-95%) of any ED treatment

- Three types of implants offer different advantages based on individual priorities
- Insurance coverage for implants is excellent when medical necessity is documented
- Constriction rings can enhance the effectiveness of other treatments
- Device based treatments work independently of vascular or nerve function
- Combination approaches often provide better results than single treatments alone

Chapter 8: Cutting-Edge Treatments

The landscape of erectile dysfunction treatment continues to evolve rapidly, with researchers exploring innovative approaches that go beyond traditional medications and devices. These emerging therapies offer hope for men who haven't achieved satisfactory results with conventional treatments, particularly those with advanced diabetes complications that make standard approaches less effective.

Understanding these cutting-edge treatments helps you make informed decisions about whether to pursue experimental options and sets realistic expectations about what's possible with current technology. While some of these approaches show tremendous promise, it's important to distinguish between treatments with solid scientific evidence and those that remain largely theoretical or unproven.

Shockwave Therapy (Li-ESWT)

Low-intensity extracorporeal shockwave therapy represents one of the most promising advances in ED treatment in the past decade. This non-invasive therapy uses focused sound waves to stimulate blood vessel growth and tissue regeneration in the penis, potentially addressing some of the root causes of diabetes-related ED rather than just treating symptoms.

How Sound Waves Restore Function

Li-ESWT works through several biological mechanisms:

Neovascularization: Sound waves stimulate the formation of new blood vessels (angiogenesis) in penile tissue, potentially bypassing damaged vessels caused by diabetes.

Tissue regeneration: The mechanical stress from sound waves activates cellular repair mechanisms and promotes healthy tissue growth.

Nerve regeneration: Some evidence suggests shockwave therapy may promote nerve healing, which could benefit men with diabetic neuropathy affecting sexual function.

Plaque disruption: In men with Peyronie's disease (penile scarring), shockwaves may help break down scar tissue.

Improved endothelial function: Treatment may restore the function of blood vessel linings, improving their ability to respond to arousal signals.

The sound waves used in Li-ESWT are the same type used to break up kidney stones, but at much lower intensity levels that don't cause tissue damage. Instead, they create beneficial stress that triggers the body's natural healing responses.

Latest 2024 Protocols by ED Severity

Treatment protocols have become more standardized as research has identified optimal parameters:

Mild ED protocol:

- 12 sessions over 6 weeks (2 sessions per week)
- 3,000 pulses per session at low intensity
- Focus areas: penile shaft, crura (roots of penis), and perineum
- Follow-up sessions at 3 and 6 months if needed

Moderate ED protocol:

- 18 sessions over 9 weeks (2 sessions per week)
- 5,000 pulses per session at moderate intensity
- More extensive treatment areas including penile base and surrounding tissues
- Potential combination with PRP therapy

Severe ED protocol:

- 24 sessions over 12 weeks (2 sessions per week)
- 6,000 pulses per session at higher intensity
- May require multiple treatment courses
- Often combined with other therapies for optimal results

Treatment Experience: Each session lasts approximately 20-30 minutes and is performed in a doctor's office. A gel is applied to the treatment area, and a handheld device delivers precisely controlled sound waves. Most men describe the sensation as mild tapping or tingling—uncomfortable but not painful.

Combination with PRP for Better Results

Many providers now combine Li-ESWT with platelet-rich plasma (PRP) therapy for enhanced results:

PRP preparation: A small amount of the patient's blood is drawn and processed to concentrate platelets and growth factors.

Injection process: PRP is injected into penile tissue either before or after shockwave treatment.

Synergistic effects: Growth factors in PRP may enhance the regenerative effects stimulated by shockwave therapy.

Improved outcomes: Combination therapy shows better results than either treatment alone in preliminary studies.

Finding Qualified Providers

Not all shockwave therapy is equal—proper equipment and technique are crucial:

Equipment requirements: Look for providers using FDA-approved devices specifically designed for erectile dysfunction treatment.

Provider experience: Choose providers with specific training in Li-ESWT for ED and a track record of successful treatments.

Treatment protocols: Ensure providers follow evidence-based protocols rather than arbitrary treatment schedules.

Outcome tracking: Quality providers track treatment responses using validated questionnaires and objective measures.

Case Example: Thomas, Age 52

Thomas, a 52-year-old engineer with Type 2 diabetes for 10 years, had moderate ED that responded poorly to oral medications. His A1C was well-controlled at 6.9%, but vascular testing showed significant penile artery disease.

"I wanted to try something that might actually fix the problem, not just treat the symptoms," Thomas explains. "The idea of using sound waves to grow new blood vessels sounded like science fiction, but the research was compelling."

Thomas underwent a comprehensive Li-ESWT protocol:

Pre-treatment evaluation: Doppler ultrasound confirmed reduced penile blood flow. IIEF score was 14 (moderate ED).

Treatment course: 18 sessions over 9 weeks, combined with PRP injections at sessions 6, 12, and 18.

Treatment experience: "The sessions were uncomfortable but not painful. It felt like someone tapping rapidly on my penis. Each session took about 25 minutes."

Results timeline:

- Month 1: No noticeable changes
- Month 2: Slightly improved morning erections
- Month 3: Better response to sildenafil
- Month 6: IIEF score improved to 19, good natural erections returning
- Month 12: IIEF score 22, excellent response to lower-dose medications

"The improvement was gradual but significant," Thomas reports. "By six months, I was having natural erections again for the first time in years. The pills worked much better too—I could use half the dose I needed before."

Follow-up testing showed measurable improvement in penile blood flow, suggesting actual tissue regeneration had occurred.

Regenerative Medicine Approaches

Regenerative medicine represents the frontier of ED treatment, aiming to restore normal erectile function by repairing or replacing damaged tissues rather than working around them.

Stem Cell Therapy Transition to Mainstream

Stem cell therapy for ED is moving from experimental to clinical practice, though it remains largely investigational:

Mechanism of action: Stem cells injected into penile tissue may differentiate into various cell types needed for erectile function, including smooth muscle cells, endothelial cells, and nerve cells.

Types of stem cells used:

- Autologous adipose-derived stem cells (from patient's own fat tissue)
- Bone marrow-derived stem cells
- Umbilical cord-derived stem cells

Treatment process: Stem cells are harvested from the patient, processed in a laboratory, then injected into specific areas of penile tissue.

Current status: Multiple clinical trials are underway, with preliminary results showing promise but long-term safety and efficacy data still being collected.

Platelet-Rich Plasma (PRP) Evidence

PRP therapy has the strongest evidence base among regenerative approaches:

Mechanism: Concentrated platelets release growth factors that promote tissue healing and blood vessel formation.

Preparation: Patient's blood is drawn and processed to concentrate platelets to 3-5 times normal levels.

Injection technique: PRP is injected into multiple sites in penile tissue under local anesthesia.

Evidence base: Several small studies show 60-70% of men experience improvement in erectile function after PRP treatment.

Safety profile: Excellent safety record since it uses the patient's own blood products.

Combination benefits: Often combined with other treatments like Li-ESWT for enhanced results.

What Insurance Covers (and Doesn't)

Most regenerative medicine approaches are not covered by insurance:

Covered treatments: Generally none, as most approaches are considered experimental.

Out-of-pocket costs:

- PRP therapy: $1,500-3,000 per treatment
- Stem cell therapy: $5,000-15,000 per treatment course
- Li-ESWT: $3,000-6,000 for complete series

Financial considerations: High costs and lack of insurance coverage limit access for many patients.

Clinical trial options: Participation in research studies may provide access to cutting-edge treatments at reduced cost.

Realistic Expectations

Setting appropriate expectations is crucial for regenerative medicine approaches:

Timeline for results: Improvements may not be apparent for 3-6 months after treatment.

Success rates: Generally 50-70% of men see some improvement, but dramatic improvements are less common.

Degree of improvement: Most men see moderate improvement rather than complete restoration of function.

Need for additional treatments: Many approaches require multiple treatment sessions for optimal results.

Combination with other therapies: Regenerative approaches often work best when combined with proven treatments.

Future Horizons

Research continues to explore increasingly sophisticated approaches to treating ED:

Gene Therapy Developments

Gene therapy aims to restore erectile function by delivering therapeutic genes directly to penile tissue:

Approaches being studied:

- Genes that promote blood vessel growth
- Genes that enhance nitric oxide production
- Genes that protect against oxidative stress and inflammation

Delivery methods: Direct injection, viral vectors, or nanoparticle delivery systems.

Current status: Preclinical and early clinical trials, with human studies still limited.

Potential advantages: Could provide long-lasting or permanent improvements with single treatments.

Challenges: Safety concerns, delivery difficulties, and regulatory hurdles.

Nanotechnology Applications

Nanotechnology offers precise ways to deliver treatments to specific tissues:

Drug delivery systems: Nanoparticles that deliver medications directly to penile tissue, potentially improving effectiveness while reducing side effects.

Tissue engineering: Nanoscale scaffolds that support tissue regeneration and blood vessel growth.

Diagnostic applications: Nanosensors that could provide real-time monitoring of erectile function and treatment response.

Current development: Mostly in research phase, with clinical applications still years away.

Personalized Medicine Approaches

The future of ED treatment may involve customized approaches based on individual genetic and molecular profiles:

Genetic testing: Identifying specific genetic factors that contribute to an individual's ED risk and treatment response.

Biomarker analysis: Using blood tests or tissue analysis to predict which treatments are most likely to work for specific patients.

Precision dosing: Adjusting medication doses based on genetic factors that affect drug metabolism.

Targeted therapies: Developing treatments aimed at specific molecular pathways involved in individual cases of ED.

Case Example: Michael, Age 46

Michael, a 46-year-old research scientist with Type 1 diabetes for 22 years, was interested in cutting-edge treatments due to his scientific background and poor response to conventional therapies.

"Having a science background, I was excited about the potential for regenerative medicine," Michael explains. "I wanted to be part of advancing treatment options, not just for myself but for other men dealing with diabetes-related ED."

Michael participated in a clinical trial combining Li-ESWT with PRP therapy:

Trial design: Randomized controlled trial comparing Li-ESWT alone versus Li-ESWT plus PRP.

Treatment protocol: 12 shockwave sessions over 6 weeks, with PRP injections at weeks 2, 4, and 6.

Monitoring: Extensive testing including Doppler ultrasound, MRI imaging, and tissue biopsies to assess treatment effects.

Results: IIEF score improved from 11 to 18 over 6 months, with objective improvements in penile blood flow.

Research contribution: Data from Michael's case and others in the trial contributed to published research advancing the field.

"Participating in research felt like the right thing to do," Michael reflects. "I got access to cutting-edge treatment, and the results were better than I expected. Knowing that my experience might help other men made it even more meaningful."

Clinical Trials You Can Join

Participating in clinical trials offers access to experimental treatments while contributing to medical knowledge:

Finding Clinical Trials: *ClinicalTrials.gov*: The official U.S. database of clinical studies. *Search terms*: "Erectile dysfunction," "diabetes," "regenerative medicine," "stem cell therapy." *Location filters*: Search by geographic area to find nearby studies.

Types of Trials Available: *Drug trials*: Testing new medications or new uses for existing drugs. *Device studies*: Evaluating new medical devices or improved versions of existing devices. *Regenerative medicine trials*: Testing stem cell therapy, PRP, or other biological treatments. *Combination therapy studies*: Evaluating combinations of existing treatments.

Eligibility Considerations: *Inclusion criteria*: Most trials require confirmed ED diagnosis, specific diabetes duration, and failure of conventional treatments. *Exclusion criteria*: Common exclusions include severe heart disease, active cancer, bleeding disorders, or use of certain medications. *Commitment requirements*: Trials typically require multiple visits over 6-12 months for treatment and follow-up.

Risks and Benefits of Participation: *Potential benefits*: Access to cutting-edge treatments, close medical monitoring, contribution to scientific knowledge. *Potential risks*: Unknown side effects, possibility of receiving placebo treatment, time commitment for visits. *Protection measures*: All trials must be approved by ethics committees and include detailed informed consent processes.

Practical Tools

New Treatment Evaluation Checklist

Before considering experimental treatments, evaluate:

Scientific evidence:

- Has the treatment been published in peer-reviewed journals?
- Are there completed clinical trials, or only preliminary studies?
- What are the reported success rates and side effects?
- How does it compare to proven treatments?

Provider qualifications:

- Does the provider have specific training in the treatment?
- Are they participating in research or just offering commercial treatments?
- Can they provide references from other patients?
- Are they transparent about costs and expected outcomes?

Cost-benefit analysis:

- What is the total cost of treatment?
- Is any portion covered by insurance?
- What are the opportunity costs of pursuing experimental treatment instead of proven options?
- Are there payment plans or financial assistance available?

Personal factors:

- Are you a good candidate based on your medical history?
- Do you have realistic expectations about outcomes?
- Are you prepared for the time commitment required?
- Have you optimized conventional treatments first?

Clinical Trial Finder Guide

Step-by-step process for finding relevant trials:

1. *Visit ClinicalTrials.gov*
2. *Search terms*: "erectile dysfunction diabetes" or "ED regenerative medicine"
3. *Filter by location*: Select your state or region
4. *Filter by status*: Choose "Recruiting" for studies currently enrolling
5. *Review eligibility*: Read inclusion/exclusion criteria carefully
6. *Contact information*: Note study coordinators' contact details
7. *Prepare questions*: List questions about time commitment, risks, and benefits

Provider Qualification Questions

Questions to ask providers offering experimental treatments:

About their experience:

- How many patients have you treated with this approach?
- What are your success rates?
- Can you provide references from other patients?
- Do you participate in research studies?

About the treatment:

- What peer-reviewed research supports this treatment?
- How does it work, and why might it help my specific situation?
- What are the potential risks and side effects?
- How will we measure success?

About costs and logistics:

- What is the total cost of treatment?
- Are there additional costs for follow-up care?
- Is any portion covered by insurance?
- What happens if the treatment doesn't work?

Treatment Diary for Emerging Therapies

Track your experience with experimental treatments:

Pre-treatment documentation:

- Baseline IIEF score
- Current medications and their effectiveness
- Specific symptoms and severity
- Goals and expectations

During treatment:

- Date and details of each session
- Side effects or reactions
- Changes in symptoms
- Questions or concerns

Post-treatment monitoring:

- Weekly symptom assessments
- Monthly IIEF scores
- Changes in response to other treatments
- Overall satisfaction and quality of life impact

The Reality Check

While emerging treatments offer exciting possibilities, it's important to maintain realistic perspectives:

What Works Now vs. What Might Work

Proven treatments: PDE5 inhibitors, injection therapy, vacuum devices, and penile implants have decades of research and clinical experience supporting their use.

Emerging treatments: Li-ESWT shows the most promise with growing evidence, while stem cell therapy and other regenerative approaches remain largely experimental.

Future treatments: Gene therapy and nanotechnology approaches are intriguing but remain years away from clinical availability.

The Importance of Proven Foundations

Before pursuing cutting-edge treatments, ensure you've optimized conventional approaches:

Diabetes control: Achieve and maintain optimal blood sugar levels. *Lifestyle factors*: Address diet, exercise, weight, sleep, and stress. *Medication optimization*: Try different PDE5 inhibitors, dosing schedules, and combinations. *Psychological factors*: Address depression, anxiety, and relationship issues.

Managing Expectations and Avoiding Scams

The desperation that ED can create makes men vulnerable to unscrupulous providers and unrealistic promises:

Red flags:

- Guarantees of success or "permanent cures"
- Pressure to pay large sums upfront
- Lack of informed consent or discussion of risks
- Providers without proper medical credentials
- Treatments not backed by published research

Protective strategies:

- Research providers thoroughly
- Seek second opinions for expensive treatments
- Ask for references from other patients
- Verify credentials and board certifications
- Be wary of treatments marketed directly to consumers

Integration with Conventional Care

The most successful approaches often combine cutting-edge treatments with proven therapies:

Combination Strategies

Li-ESWT + PDE5 inhibitors: Shockwave therapy may restore some natural function while medications provide immediate symptom relief.

PRP + injection therapy: Regenerative treatments may improve tissue health while injections provide reliable function.

Stem cell therapy + lifestyle optimization: Biological treatments may work better in the context of optimal diabetes control and cardiovascular health.

Timing Considerations

Sequential approach: Try proven treatments first, then add experimental approaches if needed. *Combination timing*: Some treatments work better when combined simultaneously rather than sequentially. *Recovery periods*: Allow adequate time between treatments to assess individual effectiveness.

The Future Is Promising

Research into ED treatment continues to accelerate, driven by better understanding of the underlying biology and advances in medical technology. Men with diabetes-related ED have reason for optimism about future treatment options.

Near-term developments (2-5 years):

- Improved shockwave therapy protocols
- Better understanding of optimal regenerative medicine approaches

- New medication formulations and delivery methods
- Enhanced combination therapy strategies

Medium-term possibilities (5-10 years):

- Gene therapy treatments for selected patients
- Tissue engineering approaches for severe cases
- Personalized medicine based on genetic profiles
- Nanotechnology-enhanced drug delivery

Long-term potential (10+ years):

- Biological restoration of normal erectile function
- Prevention strategies for high-risk individuals
- Artificial intelligence-guided treatment selection
- Revolutionary approaches we haven't yet imagined

Making Informed Decisions

The key to navigating emerging treatments is balancing optimism with realism:

Consider experimental treatments if:

- Conventional treatments have been optimized and found inadequate
- You understand the experimental nature and associated uncertainties
- The financial cost is manageable without compromising other healthcare needs
- You're prepared for the possibility that treatment may not work

Stick with proven treatments if:

- Conventional approaches haven't been fully optimized
- Experimental treatments involve significant financial hardship
- You're not comfortable with uncertainty about outcomes

- Proven treatments are providing adequate results

Questions for Decision-Making:

- Have I truly optimized all conventional treatment options?
- Do I understand the evidence base for this experimental treatment?
- Am I prepared emotionally and financially for the possibility of treatment failure?
- What are my alternatives if this approach doesn't work?

Cutting-edge treatments represent hope and possibility, but they work best in the context of comprehensive care that includes proven approaches. The men who achieve the best outcomes are those who combine evidence-based treatments with carefully selected innovative approaches, all while maintaining excellent diabetes control and overall health.

Remember that the goal isn't to be on the cutting edge for its own sake—it's to achieve satisfying sexual function using whatever combination of approaches works best for your specific situation. Sometimes that includes experimental treatments, and sometimes proven approaches provide everything you need.

The next section will shift focus from medical treatments to the equally important aspects of relationships and communication, exploring how to navigate the emotional and interpersonal challenges that diabetes-related ED creates.

Key Insights on Emerging Treatments:

- Li-ESWT shows the most promise among emerging treatments, with growing evidence of effectiveness
- Regenerative medicine approaches like PRP and stem cell therapy are promising but remain largely experimental
- Most cutting-edge treatments are not covered by insurance and require significant out-of-pocket investment
- Clinical trials offer access to experimental treatments while contributing to medical knowledge

- Combination approaches often work better than single treatments alone
- Proven treatments should be optimized before pursuing experimental options
- Future developments in gene therapy and nanotechnology offer long-term hope
- Realistic expectations and careful provider selection are crucial for experimental treatments

Chapter 9: Talking to Your Partner

One of the most challenging aspects of dealing with diabetes-related erectile dysfunction isn't the medical treatment—it's the conversation with your partner. Many men struggle in silence for months or years, allowing ED to create distance and misunderstanding in their relationships. This silence often causes more damage than the ED itself, leading to decreased intimacy, increased tension, and sometimes relationship breakdown.

Your partner can be your greatest ally in overcoming ED, but only if they understand what's happening and how they can help. Open, honest communication about sexual health challenges strengthens relationships and dramatically improves treatment outcomes. This chapter provides practical scripts and strategies for having these difficult conversations, addressing your partner's concerns, and maintaining intimacy throughout your treatment journey.

Starting the Conversation

The first conversation about ED is often the hardest, but it's also the most important. How you approach this discussion sets the tone for how you'll handle this challenge together.

When and Where to Talk

Timing considerations:

- Choose a time when you're both relaxed and won't be interrupted
- Avoid bringing it up immediately before, during, or after sexual activity
- Don't wait for a crisis moment—address it when things are calm
- Consider having the conversation during a walk or car ride if direct eye contact feels too intense

Setting considerations:

- Private space where you feel comfortable speaking openly
- Turn off phones and other distractions
- Comfortable seating where you can face each other
- Neutral location, not the bedroom where sexual pressure might be felt

Opening Scripts That Reduce Anxiety

Starting the conversation is often the hardest part. Here are several approaches that have worked for many couples:

The direct approach: "I need to talk to you about something that's been bothering me. I've been having some problems with erections, and I think it's related to my diabetes. I wanted you to know what's going on and get your thoughts on how we should handle it."

The relationship-focused approach: "I've noticed we haven't been as intimate lately, and I want you to know it's not because I'm not attracted to you. I've been dealing with some erectile problems that I think are connected to my diabetes, and I wasn't sure how to bring it up."

The team approach: "We've always been good at working through challenges together, and I'm hoping we can tackle this one too. I've been struggling with erectile dysfunction, and I'd like us to figure out the best way to address it as a couple."

The vulnerability approach: "This is really hard for me to talk about, but I trust you and need your support. I've been having trouble with erections, and it's been affecting how I feel about myself and our relationship."

What Partners Need to Hear

Your partner needs specific information and reassurance to process this news constructively:

It's medical, not personal: "This is a medical condition related to my diabetes, not anything you've done or a reflection of how I feel about you."

You're still attracted to them: "My feelings for you haven't changed at all. I'm still completely attracted to you and want to be intimate with you."

It's treatable: "There are lots of good treatment options available now, and most men with diabetes-related ED can find something that works."

You want their partnership: "I don't want to deal with this alone. I'd like us to work through this together and find solutions that work for both of us."

You're committed to the relationship: "This doesn't change my commitment to you or our relationship. If anything, I want to address it so we can be even closer."

Case Example: James, Age 48

James, a 48-year-old accountant with Type 2 diabetes for six years, had been avoiding intimacy with his wife Carol for nearly eight months. The tension in their 18-year marriage was becoming unbearable.

"I kept thinking it would get better on its own, or that maybe she hadn't noticed," James admits. "But I could see her getting more and more hurt and confused. She started asking if I was having an affair."

James finally initiated the conversation during a weekend morning when their teenage children were still sleeping:

"Carol, I need to tell you something, and it's really hard for me to talk about. You've been asking if everything's okay between us, and the truth is, I've been having problems with erections. I think it's related to my diabetes, and I've been too embarrassed to say anything."

122

Carol's initial response was relief: "I thought you weren't attracted to me anymore. I was starting to wonder if there was someone else."

James continued: "It has nothing to do with you. I'm still completely attracted to you. I just haven't known how to handle this or what to do about it. I was hoping it would go away, but it's not getting better."

"The conversation was emotional, but it was such a relief to finally be honest," James reflects. "Carol was incredibly supportive once she understood what was happening."

The couple scheduled a doctor's appointment together within a week, and James began treatment with excellent results. "Talking about it was the hardest part," Carol says. "Once we could discuss it openly, everything else felt manageable."

Addressing Common Partner Concerns

Partners often have predictable concerns and questions when they learn about ED. Anticipating and addressing these concerns helps facilitate productive conversations.

"Is it me?" - Removing Blame

This is often the first concern partners express, especially if there's been a period of avoiding intimacy:

Why partners think this: Decreased sexual activity, avoided intimacy, and changed behavior can make partners feel rejected or unattractive.

How to address it: "I understand why you might think that, especially since I've been distant lately. But this is definitely not about you or my feelings for you. ED is a known complication of diabetes that affects the blood vessels and nerves, not my attraction or love for you."

Provide education: "Would you like to come with me to talk to the doctor about this? It might help to hear from a medical professional that this is a common diabetes complication that has nothing to do with our relationship."

Reassure with actions: Continue non-sexual physical affection, compliments, and intimate conversation to reinforce that the problem is medical, not relational.

"Will this get better?" - Realistic Hope

Partners need honest information about prognosis and treatment options:

Provide realistic optimism: "The good news is that there are lots of effective treatments available now. Most men with diabetes-related ED can find something that works, though it might take some time to figure out the best approach for me."

Explain the process: "Treatment often involves trying different approaches - lifestyle changes, medications, devices, or combinations of treatments. It may take a few months to find what works best, but the success rates are very good."

Set timeline expectations: "I'd like to see a doctor within the next few weeks to start the process. Some treatments work quickly, others take longer, but we should start seeing progress within a few months."

Emphasize partnership: "I'd really like you to be involved in this process if you're comfortable with that. Your support and input will help me make the best decisions about treatment."

"How can I help?" - Concrete Actions

Partners often want to help but don't know how. Providing specific ways they can support you makes them feel useful and strengthens your partnership:

Medical support: "It would really help if you could come with me to doctor appointments. Having you there to ask questions and help me remember information would be great."

Emotional support: "Just knowing you understand that this is medical and not personal is incredibly helpful. When I'm feeling frustrated or embarrassed about this, reminding me that it doesn't change how you feel about me really helps."

Practical support: "If we decide to try treatments like vacuum devices or injections, your patience while I learn to use them properly would mean a lot. And helping me stick to lifestyle changes like diet and exercise would be amazing."

Intimacy support: "I don't want this to completely disrupt our physical intimacy. Maybe we can explore other ways to be close while I'm working on treatment options."

Maintaining Connection

ED can create a downward spiral where decreased sexual activity leads to decreased physical intimacy overall, which then affects emotional connection. Breaking this cycle requires intentional effort to maintain connection in multiple ways.

Daily Intimacy Without Pressure

Physical touch: Maintain non-sexual physical contact through hugging, hand-holding, kissing, cuddling, and casual touching throughout the day.

Emotional intimacy: Share thoughts, feelings, experiences, and daily events. Ask about your partner's day, feelings, and concerns.

Quality time: Spend focused time together without distractions like phones, TV, or work. This could be meals together, walks, or conversations.

Appreciation: Express gratitude for your partner and acknowledge things you appreciate about them and the relationship.

Non-Verbal Communication Strategies

When words feel difficult, non-verbal communication can maintain connection:

Eye contact: Maintain loving eye contact during conversations and throughout the day.

Facial expressions: Smile, show affection, and express warmth through your expressions.

Body language: Open, welcoming posture that invites closeness rather than defensive or withdrawn positioning.

Gestures: Small gestures like bringing coffee, leaving notes, or doing thoughtful things communicate care and attention.

Rebuilding Physical Touch Gradually

Start with non-sexual touch: Reestablish comfort with physical contact through cuddling, massage, and affectionate touching.

Communicate during touch: Talk about what feels good, what you're comfortable with, and what you'd like to try.

Focus on pleasure, not performance: Emphasize enjoying physical connection rather than achieving specific sexual goals.

Be patient with progress: Allow intimacy to rebuild gradually rather than trying to return to previous patterns immediately.

Case Example: Robert, Age 54

Robert, a 54-year-old construction supervisor with Type 2 diabetes for nine years, and his wife Linda had seen their physical intimacy decline dramatically over two years as Robert's ED worsened.

"We went from a very affectionate, physically close couple to barely touching," Linda explains. "Robert would tense up whenever I tried to be affectionate because he was worried it would lead to sexual expectations he couldn't meet."

After Robert's ED diagnosis and the beginning of treatment, the couple worked on rebuilding intimacy gradually:

Week 1-2: Focused on non-sexual physical contact - hand-holding during TV watching, hugging when greeting and saying goodbye, cuddling without sexual expectations.

Week 3-4: Added sensual touching like back rubs and foot massages, with clear agreements that these wouldn't lead to sexual activity.

Week 5-6: Began exploring sexual touching and intimacy without pressure for intercourse, focusing on giving and receiving pleasure.

Week 7-8: As Robert's medical treatment began showing results, gradually reintroduced intercourse with reduced performance pressure.

"The key was taking the pressure off," Robert explains. "Once we could touch and be intimate without me worrying about whether I could perform, everything got easier."

Linda adds: "We actually became more affectionate than we'd been in years. Having to rebuild intimacy intentionally made us pay attention to things we'd been taking for granted."

Practical Tools

Conversation Starter Cards

Keep these phrases available for initiating difficult conversations:

For initial disclosure:

- "I've been dealing with something that's affecting our relationship, and I want to be honest with you about it."

- "There's something medical going on that I think you should know about."
- "I need your support with a health challenge I've been facing."

For ongoing discussions:

- "How are you feeling about everything we've discussed?"
- "What questions do you have about my treatment options?"
- "Is there anything I can do to help you feel more comfortable with this situation?"

For difficult moments:

- "I know this is frustrating for both of us. How can we work through this together?"
- "I'm feeling embarrassed about this. Can you help me remember that it's not my fault?"
- "This is harder than I expected. Can we talk about how we're both handling it?"

Partner Education Handout

Information to share with your partner about diabetes-related ED:

Basic facts:

- ED affects 35-90% of men with diabetes
- It's caused by blood vessel and nerve damage from high blood sugar
- It's a medical condition, not a psychological or relationship problem
- Treatment options are numerous and effective

What to expect:

- Treatment may involve trying different approaches
- Improvement often takes time and patience
- Some treatments require partner involvement or understanding
- Open communication improves treatment success

How partners can help:

- Provide emotional support and understanding
- Participate in medical appointments when appropriate
- Maintain physical intimacy in non-sexual ways
- Be patient with treatment processes and timelines

Couple's Communication Exercises

Daily check-ins: Spend 10 minutes each day sharing how you're feeling about your relationship, treatment progress, and any concerns.

Weekly planning: Schedule time each week to discuss upcoming medical appointments, treatment decisions, or relationship goals.

Monthly evaluation: Once a month, assess progress in both medical treatment and relationship satisfaction, adjusting approaches as needed.

Gratitude practice: Regularly express appreciation for each other's efforts and support throughout the ED treatment process.

Intimacy Rebuilding Timeline

Week 1-2: Foundation building

- Increase non-sexual physical contact
- Express verbal appreciation and affection
- Spend quality time together without distractions
- Begin open communication about ED and feelings

Week 3-4: Physical comfort

- Add sensual but non-sexual touching
- Practice giving and receiving pleasure without performance pressure
- Continue building emotional intimacy through conversation
- Establish agreements about sexual expectations

Week 5-6: Sexual exploration

- Begin sexual touching and intimacy
- Focus on pleasure rather than performance
- Communicate openly about what feels good
- Maintain no-pressure environment

Week 7-8: Integration

- Gradually reintroduce intercourse as appropriate
- Continue emphasis on mutual pleasure
- Celebrate progress and successful experiences
- Develop long-term intimacy maintenance strategies

Special Considerations

For Long-Term Relationships

Couples who have been together for many years may face unique challenges:

Established patterns: Long-standing sexual routines may need to be modified or expanded.

Communication styles: Couples who haven't discussed sexual issues openly may need to develop new communication skills.

Life stage factors: Other aging-related changes may complicate the picture.

Solution strategies: Focus on rediscovering each other, be willing to try new approaches, and consider couples counseling if communication proves difficult.

For New Relationships

Men entering new relationships while dealing with ED face different challenges:

Disclosure timing: When and how to tell a new partner about ED.

Trust building: Developing enough trust to have vulnerable conversations.

Performance anxiety: New relationship pressure combined with ED anxiety.

Solution strategies: Be honest early in physical relationships, focus on building emotional intimacy first, and communicate openly about needs and concerns.

For Partners with Their Own Health Issues

When both partners have health challenges, coordination becomes important:

Competing medical needs: Balancing multiple health conditions and treatments.

Energy limitations: Managing fatigue and physical limitations from various conditions.

Medication interactions: Ensuring treatments don't interfere with each other.

Solution strategies: Coordinate medical care, communicate about energy levels and capabilities, and adapt intimacy to accommodate both partners' needs.

When Professional Help Is Needed

Sometimes couples need additional support beyond what they can provide each other:

Relationship Counseling Indicators:

- Persistent communication difficulties

- Blame or resentment that doesn't resolve with discussion
- Significant decrease in relationship satisfaction
- Disagreement about treatment approaches or priorities

Sex Therapy Benefits:

- Professional guidance for sexual communication
- Techniques for maintaining intimacy during treatment
- Strategies for adapting sexual practices
- Support for both partners' emotional needs

Finding Qualified Help:

- Look for licensed therapists with specific training in sexual health
- Ask for referrals from your healthcare providers
- Consider therapists who understand medical sexual dysfunction
- Verify credentials and experience with diabetes-related issues

Building Stronger Relationships

Many couples find that successfully navigating ED together actually strengthens their relationship:

Enhanced Communication: Learning to discuss sexual health openly often improves communication in other areas.

Deeper Intimacy: Working through challenges together can create stronger emotional bonds.

Greater Appreciation: Overcoming obstacles often increases gratitude for the relationship.

Improved Problem-Solving: Successfully addressing ED builds confidence for handling future challenges.

Renewed Romance: Intentionally rebuilding intimacy can rekindle romance and appreciation.

The key to success is approaching ED as a challenge you face together rather than a problem one partner has that affects the other. When couples unite in addressing ED, they often emerge with stronger, more intimate relationships than they had before.

Essential Communication Insights:

- Early, honest communication about ED prevents misunderstanding and relationship damage
- Partners need specific reassurance that ED is medical, not personal or relational
- Providing concrete ways partners can help makes them feel useful and strengthens partnership
- Maintaining non-sexual intimacy is crucial while addressing sexual function
- Gradual rebuilding of physical intimacy works better than trying to return to previous patterns immediately
- Professional help is beneficial when couples struggle with communication or adaptation
- Successfully navigating ED together often strengthens relationships long-term
- The goal is partnership in addressing challenges, not one person fixing a problem alone

Chapter 10: Redefining Intimacy

The cultural narrative around male sexuality often reduces satisfying sex to one simple equation: erection plus penetration equals success. This narrow definition becomes a trap for men dealing with erectile dysfunction, creating performance pressure that can worsen the problem and limiting the possibilities for pleasurable, intimate sexual experiences.

Redefining intimacy beyond penetration isn't about settling for less—it's about discovering more. Many couples find that expanding their definition of satisfying sex leads to greater variety, deeper connection, and more consistent pleasure than they experienced when focused solely on penetrative intercourse. This shift in perspective can reduce performance anxiety, increase sexual confidence, and create a foundation for sexual satisfaction that doesn't depend entirely on erectile function.

The Pleasure Priority Shift

The first step in redefining intimacy involves shifting focus from performance to pleasure, from goals to experiences, and from individual function to mutual satisfaction.

Why Penetration Isn't Everything

The emphasis on penetrative sex as the ultimate sexual experience is largely cultural rather than biological:

Historical perspective: Many cultures throughout history have valued various forms of sexual expression equally, not prioritizing penetration above all else.

Physiological reality: The most sensitive parts of both male and female genitals are often not those most stimulated during penetrative intercourse.

Pleasure research: Studies consistently show that many women achieve more reliable and intense orgasms through clitoral stimulation than through penetration alone.

Variety benefits: Sexual experiences that include multiple types of stimulation and connection often lead to greater satisfaction for both partners.

Pressure reduction: When penetration becomes one option among many rather than the required goal, performance anxiety decreases significantly.

What Partners Really Want (Research Data)

Research on sexual satisfaction reveals that partners value many aspects of intimate connection beyond penetrative intercourse:

Emotional connection: Studies consistently show that feeling emotionally connected to one's partner is the strongest predictor of sexual satisfaction.

Attention and presence: Partners value feeling that their partner is fully present and focused during intimate moments.

Variety and creativity: Sexual experiences that include variety and novelty are associated with higher satisfaction levels.

Communication: Partners who communicate openly about preferences and desires report higher sexual satisfaction.

Non-goal-oriented pleasure: Sexual experiences focused on mutual pleasure rather than specific outcomes (like orgasm) often lead to greater satisfaction.

Whole-body intimacy: Touch, kissing, caressing, and sensual contact throughout the body contribute significantly to sexual satisfaction.

Permission to Explore

Many couples have never given themselves permission to explore sexual options beyond traditional intercourse:

Cultural messaging: Societal messages often suggest that "real sex" requires penetration, limiting couples' exploration of alternatives.

Relationship habits: Long-term relationships may fall into routine patterns that haven't been questioned or expanded.

Educational limitations: Many people haven't been exposed to information about the full range of pleasurable sexual activities.

Performance pressure: The focus on erectile function may have prevented exploration of activities that don't require erections.

Communication barriers: Couples may not have discussed their interests in different types of sexual activity.

Giving yourself and your partner permission to explore beyond penetration opens up a world of possibilities for intimate connection and mutual pleasure.

Expanding Your Repertoire

Developing a broader range of intimate activities requires both knowledge and willingness to experiment. The goal is to build a menu of options that provide pleasure and connection regardless of erectile function.

Sensate Focus Exercises

Sensate focus is a series of structured touching exercises developed by sex therapists to help couples reconnect with physical pleasure without performance pressure:

Stage 1: Non-genital touching

- Partners take turns touching each other's bodies, excluding genitals and breasts
- Focus is on the sensations of touching and being touched, not on arousal
- No expectations for sexual response or orgasm
- Sessions typically last 15-20 minutes per person

Stage 2: Genital touching without pressure

- Includes genital and breast touching but without goals of arousal or orgasm
- Continue focusing on sensation and pleasure rather than response
- Maintain the non-demand, exploratory approach
- Communication about preferences is encouraged

Stage 3: Mutual touching with arousal

- Both partners can touch simultaneously
- Arousal and orgasm are permitted but not required
- Maintain focus on pleasure and connection
- Transition to more interactive intimate contact

Benefits of sensate focus:

- Reduces performance anxiety by removing goals and expectations
- Helps partners rediscover physical pleasure and connection
- Improves communication about preferences and desires
- Builds confidence in intimate situations
- Creates positive sexual experiences independent of erectile function

Oral and Manual Techniques

Developing skill and comfort with oral and manual stimulation expands options for mutual pleasure:

For giving pleasure to female partners:

- Clitoral stimulation techniques using fingers, tongue, or toys
- G-spot stimulation through manual techniques
- Combination approaches using multiple types of stimulation
- Communication about pressure, rhythm, and preferences

For receiving pleasure as a male partner:

- Oral stimulation techniques that feel good regardless of firmness
- Manual stimulation that can be pleasurable even without full erection
- Exploring different areas of sensitivity beyond just the penis
- Communicating about what feels good and what to avoid

General principles:

- Start slowly and build intensity gradually
- Pay attention to partner's responses and feedback
- Vary techniques, pressure, and rhythm
- Use lubrication when helpful
- Focus on the journey rather than the destination

Using Aids and Toys Effectively

Sex toys and aids can enhance pleasure and provide options when erectile function is limited:

Vibrators: Can provide intense stimulation for female partners and may also be enjoyable for male partners.

Couples' toys: Designed to be used during intercourse or other partnered activities.

Massage oils and warming lubricants: Enhance sensation and comfort during intimate touching.

Cock rings: May help maintain erections when some erectile function exists.

Strap-on devices: Can provide penetration options when desired, regardless of erectile function.

Guidelines for toy use:

- Choose body-safe materials (silicone, glass, stainless steel)
- Start with smaller, less intimidating options
- Use appropriate lubricants
- Clean toys thoroughly between uses
- Communicate about comfort and preferences

The "Shallowing" Technique

When some erectile function exists but isn't sufficient for deep penetration, the shallowing technique can provide pleasurable contact:

Technique description: Involves shallow penetration or contact with the vulva area using a partially erect penis.

Benefits: Provides intimate contact and pleasure for both partners without requiring full erection.

Variations: Can be combined with manual or toy stimulation for additional pleasure.

Communication: Requires open discussion about what feels good and what doesn't work.

Case Example: Martin, Age 51

Martin, a 51-year-old teacher with Type 2 diabetes for seven years, and his wife Elena had been married for 24 years when Martin's ED began affecting their sexual relationship. Initially, they tried to continue their established sexual routine, leading to frustration and decreased intimacy.

"We had gotten into a pretty standard pattern over the years," Martin explains. "Elena would come to bed, we'd kiss for a few minutes, then move to intercourse. When that stopped working, we just... stopped."

Elena adds: "It felt awkward to try anything different. We'd been together so long that changing our routine felt weird, even though what we were doing wasn't working anymore."

Working with a sex therapist, Martin and Elena began exploring expanded intimacy:

Sensate focus exercises: "At first it felt artificial, like homework," Elena admits. "But after a few sessions, we started really paying attention to touch and sensation in ways we hadn't in years."

Extended foreplay: "We discovered that spending longer on kissing, touching, and oral stimulation was actually more satisfying than our old routine," Martin says.

Toy introduction: "Elena was initially hesitant about using toys, but when we found ones that enhanced pleasure for both of us, it became fun rather than clinical."

Communication improvement: "We started talking about what we liked and wanted to try. We'd never really done that in 24 years of marriage," Elena reflects.

Results after six months:

- Reported sexual satisfaction improved significantly for both partners
- Frequency of sexual activity increased compared to before ED
- Martin's performance anxiety decreased substantially
- Elena experienced more consistent orgasms than in previous years
- Overall relationship satisfaction improved

"The irony is that our sex life got better after Martin developed ED," Elena explains. "We had to learn new things and communicate more, and it turns out that made everything more exciting and satisfying."

Building New Sexual Confidence

Confidence in sexual situations doesn't have to depend on erectile function. Building confidence around expanded definitions of sexuality creates a foundation for long-term sexual satisfaction.

Reframing "Success"

Traditional definitions of sexual success often center on male performance and specific outcomes. Reframing success around mutual pleasure and connection creates more achievable and satisfying goals:

Old framework: Success = erection + penetration + male orgasm *New framework*: Success = mutual pleasure + emotional connection + satisfaction for both partners

Performance-based goals: Duration of intercourse, firmness of erection, multiple orgasms *Pleasure-based goals*: Feeling connected, experiencing pleasure, enjoying the process

Individual achievement: "I need to perform well" *Mutual experience*: "We create pleasure together"

Outcome-focused: "Did we have 'real' sex?" *Process-focused*: "Did we enjoy our intimate time together?"

Celebrating Small Wins

Building sexual confidence requires recognizing and celebrating progress rather than focusing on limitations:

Examples of wins to celebrate:

141

- Successful intimate touching without performance pressure
- Open communication about desires and preferences
- Positive sexual experiences regardless of erectile function
- Increased comfort with new techniques or activities
- Improved emotional connection during intimate moments

Recognition strategies:

- Verbally acknowledge good experiences with your partner
- Keep a private journal of positive sexual experiences
- Focus on what worked well rather than what didn't
- Express gratitude for your partner's patience and exploration
- Celebrate relationship improvements alongside sexual improvements

Creating New Sexual Scripts

Sexual scripts are the mental models we use to understand how sexual encounters "should" unfold. Creating new scripts that don't require specific erectile function allows for more flexible and satisfying experiences:

Traditional script:

1. Brief foreplay/arousal building
2. Male erection achievement
3. Penetrative intercourse
4. Male orgasm ending the encounter

Expanded script options:

1. Extended sensual touching and connection
2. Varied types of stimulation for both partners
3. Multiple forms of pleasure and intimacy
4. Satisfaction for both partners through various means
5. Connection and aftercare regardless of specific activities

Script flexibility:

- Different approaches for different moods and circumstances
- Adaptation based on current erectile function
- Emphasis on what's possible rather than what's not
- Responsiveness to both partners' needs and desires

Practical Tools

Sensate Focus Progression Guide

Week 1-2: Non-genital touching

- 15-20 minutes per partner
- Focus on back, arms, legs, neck, feet
- No genital or breast contact
- Communicate about pressure, technique, preferences
- Goal: Rediscover non-sexual touch pleasure

Week 3-4: Genital touching without goals

- Include genital and breast touching
- No pressure for arousal or orgasm
- Continue focus on sensation and exploration
- Maintain communication about preferences
- Goal: Become comfortable with genital touch without performance pressure

Week 5-6: Mutual touching with arousal

- Both partners can touch simultaneously
- Arousal and orgasm permitted but not required
- Explore what feels good for both partners
- Begin integrating learned preferences
- Goal: Create positive, low-pressure sexual experiences

Pleasure Mapping Exercises

Individual exploration:

- Spend time exploring your own body to understand what feels good
- Note areas of sensitivity and preferred types of touch
- Practice self-stimulation techniques that don't require full erection
- Develop awareness of pleasure independent of performance

Partner exploration:

- Take turns exploring each other's bodies with curious, non-goal-oriented touch
- Ask questions about preferences and comfort
- Try different types of pressure, rhythm, and technique
- Map out what brings pleasure to each partner

Communication during exploration:

- Use specific language about what feels good
- Give feedback about pressure, speed, and technique
- Express appreciation for willingness to explore
- Discuss discoveries and preferences openly

Toy Selection Guide

For beginners:

- Start with smaller, less intimidating options
- Choose high-quality, body-safe materials
- Consider multipurpose toys that can be used in various ways
- Read reviews and educational materials before purchasing

Types to consider:

- Vibrators for external stimulation
- Couples' rings that can be used during various activities
- Massage oils and lubricants for enhanced sensation
- Small, non-intimidating internal toys

Shopping tips:

- Buy from reputable retailers that provide education and support
- Consider online shopping for privacy and better selection
- Look for toys with good warranties and customer support
- Start with one item and expand gradually based on experience

New Intimacy Ideas Generator

Sensual activities:

- Full-body massage with oils or lotions
- Sensual feeding of favorite foods
- Dancing together, clothed or unclothed
- Bathing or showering together
- Reading erotic literature aloud

Exploration activities:

- Trying new locations for intimacy
- Exploring different times of day for sexual activity
- Experimenting with different types of touch and pressure
- Playing games that involve intimate touching or communication
- Creating romantic, intimate environments

Communication activities:

- Sharing sexual fantasies or desires
- Discussing favorite past sexual experiences
- Planning future intimate experiences together
- Expressing appreciation for each other's efforts and openness
- Setting goals for sexual exploration and intimacy

Addressing Common Concerns

"This Doesn't Feel Like 'Real' Sex"

Many people struggle with expanding their definition of sex beyond penetration:

Acknowledge the feeling: It's normal to feel this way initially, given cultural messaging about what constitutes "real" sex.

Challenge the assumption: Ask why penetration is more "real" than other forms of mutual sexual pleasure and intimate connection.

Focus on outcomes: If the goal is mutual pleasure, connection, and satisfaction, many activities can achieve this effectively.

Give it time: Comfort with expanded sexuality often develops gradually as positive experiences accumulate.

"My Partner Will Be Disappointed"

Concerns about partner satisfaction are common but often unfounded:

Communicate directly: Ask your partner about their preferences and satisfaction rather than making assumptions.

Focus on their pleasure: Many partners appreciate increased attention to their pleasure and satisfaction.

Recognize the opportunity: Expanding sexual repertoire often leads to discoveries about what partners particularly enjoy.

Trust their words: When partners express satisfaction with new approaches, believe them rather than doubting their honesty.

"I Feel Less Masculine"

Traditional concepts of masculinity can interfere with accepting expanded sexuality:

Redefine masculine sexuality: True masculine confidence comes from being able to pleasure and satisfy your partner, regardless of the specific methods used.

Focus on skills: Developing expertise in various forms of pleasuring can enhance rather than diminish masculine confidence.

Consider partner perspective: Partners often find men who are attentive to their pleasure and willing to explore more attractive and masculine.

Seek support: Talking to other men who have navigated similar challenges can provide perspective and encouragement.

Long-Term Benefits

Couples who successfully expand their intimate repertoire often experience benefits that extend beyond addressing ED:

Enhanced Communication: Learning to discuss sexual preferences openly improves communication in all areas of the relationship.

Increased Variety: Having more options for intimate connection prevents sexual routines from becoming boring or repetitive.

Reduced Performance Pressure: When multiple options exist for satisfying sexual experiences, pressure on any single aspect decreases.

Greater Intimacy: Extended exploration and communication often deepen emotional connection between partners.

Improved Problem-Solving: Successfully adapting to challenges builds confidence for handling future difficulties.

Renewed Excitement: Discovering new aspects of sexuality can rekindle excitement and passion in long-term relationships.

The Path to Sexual Freedom

Redefining intimacy beyond penetration isn't about accepting limitations—it's about discovering freedom. Freedom from narrow definitions of sexual success, freedom from performance anxiety, and freedom to explore the full range of human sexual expression and connection.

This expanded approach to sexuality often leads to greater satisfaction, more consistent pleasure, and deeper intimacy than couples experienced when focused solely on traditional intercourse. It creates a foundation for sexual satisfaction that can adapt to changing health conditions, aging, and life circumstances.

The journey requires openness, communication, and patience, but the rewards extend far beyond addressing erectile dysfunction. Many couples find that this challenge becomes an opportunity to develop a richer, more satisfying sexual relationship than they ever thought possible.

Core Principles for Intimate Success:

- Sexual satisfaction doesn't require penetration—it requires connection, communication, and mutual pleasure
- Expanding sexual repertoire often leads to greater satisfaction than traditional approaches alone
- Performance anxiety decreases when multiple options exist for pleasurable intimate experiences
- Partners often value attention, presence, and creativity more than specific sexual functions
- Sensate focus exercises can rebuild intimate connection without performance pressure
- Communication about preferences and desires is essential for developing satisfying alternatives
- Building new sexual confidence requires reframing success around mutual pleasure rather than individual performance
- Long-term benefits of expanded intimacy extend throughout the relationship, not just sexual experiences

Chapter 11: Mental Health and Masculinity

The psychological impact of diabetes-related erectile dysfunction extends far beyond sexual function. For many men, ED challenges fundamental beliefs about masculinity, self-worth, and identity. The combination of managing a chronic disease like diabetes and dealing with sexual dysfunction can create a perfect storm of anxiety, depression, and diminished self-esteem that actually worsens erectile problems and impairs overall quality of life.

Understanding and addressing the mental health aspects of ED isn't optional—it's essential for successful treatment and long-term well-being. This chapter explores the psychological challenges that diabetes-related ED creates, provides tools for rebuilding healthy self-concept, and guides you toward professional resources that can accelerate your recovery.

Breaking the Performance Trap

The performance trap is a vicious cycle where anxiety about sexual function creates physiological responses that worsen erectile dysfunction, which then increases anxiety, creating an escalating spiral of sexual and psychological distress.

Why Anxiety Makes ED Worse

The relationship between anxiety and erectile function is both psychological and physiological:

Stress hormone effects: Anxiety triggers the release of adrenaline and cortisol, which constrict blood vessels and interfere with the relaxation necessary for erections.

Nervous system interference: The sympathetic nervous system activation that occurs during anxiety directly opposes the parasympathetic nervous system activity required for erectile function.

Cognitive distraction: Worrying about performance during sexual activity prevents the mental focus and presence necessary for natural arousal.

Muscle tension: Anxiety creates physical tension that interferes with the blood flow and relaxation necessary for erections.

Anticipatory anxiety: Once ED occurs, fear of future episodes can create anxiety that makes subsequent episodes more likely.

The result is a self-reinforcing cycle: ED creates anxiety, anxiety worsens ED, which increases anxiety, and so on. Breaking this cycle requires addressing both the psychological and physical aspects of the problem.

Cognitive Restructuring Techniques

Cognitive restructuring involves identifying and changing negative thought patterns that contribute to performance anxiety:

Identifying cognitive distortions:

- Catastrophizing: "If I can't get an erection, I'm not a real man"
- All-or-nothing thinking: "If the sex isn't perfect, it's a complete failure"
- Mind reading: "My partner is disappointed and thinking about leaving me"
- Fortune telling: "This will never get better, and my relationship is doomed"

Challenging negative thoughts:

- Evidence examination: "What evidence do I have that this thought is true?"
- Alternative perspectives: "What are other ways to look at this situation?"
- Realistic assessment: "How likely is this worst-case scenario actually?"

- Helpful vs. harmful: "Is this thought helping me or making things worse?"

Developing balanced thoughts:

- Instead of: "I failed as a man"
- Try: "I'm dealing with a medical condition that affects sexual function"
- Instead of: "My partner will leave me"
- Try: "My partner has been supportive, and we can work through this together"
- Instead of: "This will never get better"
- Try: "Treatment takes time, and many men find solutions that work"

Mindfulness for Sexual Health

Mindfulness practices can help break the performance anxiety cycle by developing present-moment awareness and reducing anxiety:

Mindful awareness during intimacy:

- Focus on physical sensations rather than performance expectations
- Notice thoughts without judgment and gently return attention to the present
- Pay attention to partner connection and mutual pleasure
- Practice acceptance of whatever happens without labeling it as success or failure

Daily mindfulness practices:

- 10-15 minutes of daily meditation to build general anxiety management skills
- Body scan exercises to develop awareness of physical tension and relaxation
- Breathing exercises to activate the parasympathetic nervous system

- Mindful movement like yoga or tai chi to connect mind and body

Specific techniques for sexual situations:

- Deep breathing before and during intimate moments
- Progressive muscle relaxation to release physical tension
- Grounding techniques using the five senses to stay present
- Self-compassion practices when performance doesn't meet expectations

Case Example: Kevin, Age 49

Kevin, a 49-year-old sales manager with Type 2 diabetes for eight years, developed severe performance anxiety after experiencing his first episodes of ED. His anxiety became so intense that he began avoiding sexual situations entirely.

"I went from occasionally having trouble with erections to being completely terrified of any sexual situation," Kevin explains. "Even when my wife just touched me affectionately, I'd start worrying about whether it might lead to sex and whether I'd be able to perform."

Kevin's anxiety manifested in multiple ways:

- Physical symptoms: rapid heartbeat, sweating, muscle tension
- Cognitive symptoms: racing thoughts, catastrophic predictions, inability to focus
- Behavioral symptoms: avoidance of intimacy, withdrawal from his wife, reluctance to seek medical help

Working with a therapist who specialized in sexual dysfunction, Kevin learned cognitive restructuring techniques:

Thought challenging: Kevin learned to identify catastrophic thoughts like "I'll never be able to satisfy my wife again" and challenge them with questions like "What evidence do I have for this?" and "What would I tell a friend in this situation?"

Mindfulness practice: Kevin began a daily meditation practice and learned to use breathing techniques during intimate moments to stay present rather than worrying about outcomes.

Gradual exposure: Kevin and his wife gradually reintroduced physical intimacy, starting with non-sexual touching and building up to sexual activity, with the agreement that there were no performance expectations.

Communication skills: Kevin learned to express his anxiety to his wife rather than withdrawing, which helped her understand his behavior and provide appropriate support.

After three months of therapy combined with medical treatment for ED:

- Kevin's performance anxiety decreased significantly
- His erectile function improved markedly when anxiety was reduced
- His relationship with his wife strengthened through improved communication
- Kevin developed confidence in handling setbacks without spiraling into catastrophic thinking

"Learning to manage my anxiety was just as important as the medical treatment," Kevin reflects. "Once I stopped being so afraid of failing, I actually started succeeding again."

Redefining What Makes a Man

Traditional concepts of masculinity often emphasize sexual performance as a core component of male identity. This narrow definition becomes problematic when medical conditions like diabetes affect sexual function, requiring a broader, healthier understanding of masculine identity.

Beyond Sexual Performance

Healthy masculinity encompasses many qualities that don't depend on erectile function:

Emotional strength: The ability to handle challenges, support others, and maintain resilience in difficult situations.

Character qualities: Integrity, kindness, reliability, honesty, and moral courage.

Relationship skills: The ability to love, support, communicate with, and care for family and friends.

Life achievements: Success in work, community involvement, personal growth, and contribution to others' lives.

Problem-solving abilities: The capacity to identify challenges and develop effective solutions.

Leadership qualities: The ability to guide, mentor, and inspire others.

Physical and mental health management: Taking responsibility for maintaining overall health and well-being.

Finding New Sources of Confidence

Building confidence beyond sexual performance requires identifying and developing other areas of strength and competence:

Professional accomplishments: Recognition and pride in work achievements, skills development, and career progress.

Relationship quality: Deep, meaningful connections with spouse, children, family, and friends.

Physical fitness: Strength, endurance, and health achievements appropriate for your age and condition.

Personal growth: Learning new skills, developing emotional intelligence, and expanding knowledge.

Community contribution: Volunteer work, mentoring others, and making positive impacts in your community.

Creative expression: Artistic pursuits, hobbies, and creative projects that provide satisfaction and accomplishment.

Spiritual development: Growth in faith, purpose, meaning, and connection to something larger than yourself.

Cultural Considerations

Different cultural backgrounds may emphasize different aspects of masculinity, requiring tailored approaches to redefining male identity:

Latino/Hispanic cultures: May emphasize family leadership, provider role, and protection of family honor.

African American culture: May focus on resilience, community leadership, and overcoming obstacles.

Asian cultures: May emphasize honor, family responsibility, and educational/professional achievement.

European American culture: May stress individual achievement, emotional control, and financial success.

Religious communities: May emphasize spiritual leadership, moral behavior, and service to others.

Understanding your cultural context helps identify which aspects of masculinity are most important to your identity and which areas might need reframing in light of ED challenges.

Professional Help That Works

While self-help strategies are valuable, professional mental health support often accelerates recovery and provides tools that are difficult to develop independently.

When to See a Therapist

Consider professional help if you experience:

Persistent depression or anxiety: Symptoms that last more than a few weeks and interfere with daily functioning.

Relationship problems: Conflict, communication difficulties, or decreased intimacy that don't improve with effort.

Avoidance behaviors: Avoiding sexual situations, social activities, or medical appointments due to ED-related anxiety.

Substance use: Increased alcohol or drug use to cope with ED-related stress.

Work or life interference: ED-related psychological distress affecting job performance, family relationships, or daily activities.

Suicidal thoughts: Any thoughts of self-harm or suicide require immediate professional attention.

Treatment resistance: When medical treatments for ED aren't working as expected, psychological factors may be interfering.

Types of Therapy for ED

Different therapeutic approaches offer various benefits for men dealing with diabetes-related ED:

Cognitive Behavioral Therapy (CBT):

- Focuses on identifying and changing negative thought patterns and behaviors
- Highly effective for anxiety and depression related to ED
- Provides concrete tools for managing performance anxiety
- Usually short-term (12-20 sessions) with specific goals

Sex Therapy:

- Specialized therapy focusing specifically on sexual dysfunction and relationships
- Includes communication skills, intimacy exercises, and sexual education
- Often involves both partners in treatment
- Addresses both psychological and relationship aspects of sexual problems

Acceptance and Commitment Therapy (ACT):

- Focuses on accepting difficult feelings while committing to valued actions
- Helps develop psychological flexibility in dealing with ED challenges
- Emphasizes living according to personal values rather than avoiding discomfort
- Particularly helpful for men struggling with acceptance of chronic health conditions

Mindfulness-Based Therapies:

- Incorporate meditation and mindfulness practices into traditional therapy
- Effective for reducing anxiety and improving sexual function
- Help develop present-moment awareness and reduce performance pressure
- Can be combined with other therapeutic approaches

Group Support Benefits

Group therapy or support groups offer unique advantages for men dealing with ED:

Normalization: Hearing other men's experiences reduces feelings of isolation and shame.

Peer support: Learning from men who have successfully addressed similar challenges.

Accountability: Group members can support each other in implementing treatment plans and lifestyle changes.

Diverse perspectives: Exposure to different approaches and solutions for similar problems.

Cost effectiveness: Group therapy typically costs less than individual therapy.

Social connection: Developing friendships with other men facing similar challenges.

Online Resources and Apps

Technology-based mental health resources can supplement or provide initial support:

Therapy apps:

- BetterHelp, Talkspace: Online therapy platforms with licensed therapists
- Headspace, Calm: Meditation and mindfulness apps
- MoodTools, Sanvello: Apps for managing depression and anxiety

Educational websites:

- Sexual Medicine Society of North America: Reliable medical information

- American Association of Sexuality Educators: Educational resources
- Men's Health Network: Resources specifically for men's health challenges

Online support groups:

- Reddit communities focused on ED and men's health
- Facebook support groups for men with diabetes
- Professional organization-sponsored online support groups

Considerations for online resources:

- Verify credentials of providers and legitimacy of platforms
- Online resources work best as supplements to, not replacements for, professional care
- Privacy and security should be carefully evaluated
- Apps and online resources vary widely in quality and evidence base

Case Example: Marcus, Age 56

Marcus, a 56-year-old police officer with Type 1 diabetes for 28 years, experienced severe depression following the onset of ED. His identity as a strong, capable protector was shattered by what he saw as a fundamental failure of his masculinity.

"I've been the guy people call when they need help," Marcus explains. "I've been a cop for 30 years, served in the military, raised three kids. But when I couldn't perform sexually, I felt like everything I thought I knew about myself was wrong."

Marcus's depression manifested as:

- Loss of interest in activities he previously enjoyed
- Withdrawal from family and social relationships
- Increased irritability and anger
- Sleep disturbances and fatigue
- Negative thoughts about his worth and future

Initially reluctant to seek help ("Real men don't need therapy"), Marcus eventually entered counseling at his wife's insistence and his supervisor's recommendation after his job performance began to suffer.

Individual therapy: Marcus worked with a therapist who specialized in men's issues and understood the culture of first responders. Therapy focused on:

- Challenging rigid concepts of masculinity that tied self-worth to sexual performance
- Identifying other sources of strength and identity
- Developing coping strategies for managing depression and anxiety
- Processing grief over physical changes related to diabetes

Group therapy: Marcus joined a support group for men dealing with health-related challenges, which included several other first responders and military veterans.

Couples therapy: Marcus and his wife attended several sessions to improve communication and rebuild intimacy.

After six months of therapy:

- Marcus's depression scores improved from severe to mild
- His relationship with his wife strengthened significantly
- He developed a broader, healthier concept of masculinity
- His work performance returned to previous high levels
- He became a mentor for other officers dealing with health challenges

"Therapy taught me that being strong sometimes means asking for help," Marcus reflects. "My worth as a man isn't determined by my erections—it's determined by how I treat people, how I handle challenges, and how I contribute to my family and community."

Practical Tools

Daily Mood and ED Tracker

Track the connection between your emotional state and sexual function:

Daily ratings (1-10 scale):

- Overall mood
- Anxiety level
- Stress level
- Energy level
- Relationship satisfaction
- Sexual confidence
- Erectile function (if sexual activity occurred)

Weekly patterns:

- Look for connections between emotional states and sexual function
- Identify triggers that worsen mood or increase anxiety
- Note activities or circumstances that improve mood and confidence

Monthly review:

- Assess progress in both emotional and sexual health
- Identify areas needing additional attention
- Celebrate improvements and positive changes

Anxiety Reduction Exercises

4-7-8 Breathing:

1. Inhale through nose for 4 counts
2. Hold breath for 7 counts
3. Exhale through mouth for 8 counts
4. Repeat 4-8 times

Progressive Muscle Relaxation:

1. Tense muscle groups for 5 seconds, then relax
2. Start with feet and work up to head
3. Notice the contrast between tension and relaxation
4. Practice daily to develop relaxation skills

Grounding Technique (5-4-3-2-1):

- 5 things you can see
- 4 things you can touch
- 3 things you can hear
- 2 things you can smell
- 1 thing you can taste

Mindful Meditation:

1. Sit comfortably and close eyes
2. Focus on breathing without changing it
3. When mind wanders, gently return to breath
4. Start with 5 minutes, gradually increase

Therapist Selection Guide

Credentials to look for:

- Licensed psychologist, licensed clinical social worker, or licensed marriage and family therapist
- Specific training in sexual dysfunction or men's issues
- Experience working with medical sexual dysfunction
- Comfort discussing sexual topics openly

Questions to ask potential therapists:

- What experience do you have treating ED and related psychological issues?
- What therapeutic approaches do you use for sexual dysfunction?
- Do you involve partners in treatment when appropriate?

- How do you coordinate with medical providers?
- What are your fees and insurance policies?

Red flags to avoid:

- Guarantees of quick fixes or cures
- Discomfort discussing sexual topics
- Lack of relevant experience or training
- Pressure to commit to long-term treatment immediately
- Unwillingness to coordinate with medical providers

Support Group Finder

Types of groups to consider:

- ED support groups (online or in-person)
- Men's health support groups
- Diabetes support groups that address complications
- General men's therapy groups
- Couples' groups for relationship challenges

Resources for finding groups:

- Psychology Today website has support group directories
- Hospital and medical center community education programs
- Urologist or endocrinologist referrals
- Mental health center community programs
- Online platforms like Meetup or Facebook groups

Evaluating group fit:

- Attend a few sessions before committing
- Ensure the group is led by a qualified professional
- Look for groups with similar demographics or challenges
- Verify that the group maintains confidentiality
- Choose groups that feel supportive rather than competitive or negative

Building Resilience

Mental health recovery isn't just about addressing problems—it's about building resilience and developing skills for handling future challenges:

Developing Emotional Intelligence

Self-awareness: Understanding your emotions, triggers, and patterns of response.

Self-regulation: Managing emotional reactions and choosing thoughtful responses rather than impulsive reactions.

Motivation: Finding internal drive and purpose that doesn't depend on external validation.

Empathy: Understanding and connecting with others' emotions and experiences.

Social skills: Building and maintaining healthy relationships through effective communication and conflict resolution.

Creating Meaning and Purpose

Value identification: Clarifying what matters most to you beyond sexual performance.

Goal setting: Developing meaningful goals related to relationships, health, work, and personal growth.

Legacy thinking: Considering the impact you want to have on others and how you want to be remembered.

Service opportunities: Finding ways to contribute to others' well-being and your community.

Spiritual exploration: Developing connection to purposes and meanings larger than yourself.

The Integrated Approach

The most successful treatment for diabetes-related ED addresses both the physical and psychological aspects simultaneously. Mental health support doesn't replace medical treatment—it enhances it by removing psychological barriers to recovery and building resilience for long-term success.

Men who address the psychological aspects of ED often find that:

- Medical treatments work more effectively
- Relationship satisfaction improves significantly
- Overall quality of life increases beyond just sexual function
- Confidence and self-esteem recover and grow stronger
- They develop skills for handling other life challenges more effectively

The journey from ED-related psychological distress to renewed confidence and healthy masculinity requires courage, patience, and often professional support. But the rewards extend far beyond sexual function to encompass overall mental health, relationship quality, and life satisfaction.

Mental Health and Recovery Essentials:

- Performance anxiety creates a vicious cycle that worsens ED both psychologically and physiologically
- Cognitive restructuring techniques can break negative thought patterns that fuel performance anxiety
- Healthy masculinity encompasses many qualities beyond sexual performance
- Professional therapy often accelerates recovery and provides tools difficult to develop independently
- Different types of therapy offer various benefits, from CBT for anxiety to sex therapy for relationship issues

- Group support provides unique benefits including normalization and peer learning
- Building resilience and emotional intelligence supports long-term recovery and life satisfaction
- Addressing psychological aspects enhances the effectiveness of medical treatments rather than replacing them

Chapter 12: Your 90-Day Action Plan

Recovery from diabetes-related erectile dysfunction doesn't happen overnight, but it also doesn't require years of uncertainty. Most men can see significant improvement within 90 days of implementing a comprehensive, systematic approach. This structured timeline helps you prioritize actions, track progress, and maintain motivation during the recovery process.

The 90-day framework divides your journey into three distinct phases: foundation building (days 1-30), treatment implementation (days 31-60), and optimization and maintenance (days 61-90). Each phase has specific goals, milestones, and adjustments that build upon previous progress while moving you steadily toward restored sexual function and improved quality of life.

Days 1-30: Foundation Building

The first month focuses on establishing the groundwork for successful ED treatment. This phase emphasizes medical evaluation, lifestyle optimization, and relationship preparation rather than expecting immediate sexual function improvements.

Medical Evaluation Checklist

Week 1 priorities:

- Schedule appointment with primary care provider or urologist
- Gather medical history documentation (diabetes duration, complications, medications)
- Compile list of all current medications and supplements
- Document sexual function history and timeline of changes
- Check insurance coverage for ED evaluation and treatments

Week 2 goals:

- Complete initial medical evaluation

- Obtain necessary laboratory tests (A1C, testosterone, lipids, PSA)
- Begin optimizing diabetes control with healthcare provider
- Review and adjust medications that might contribute to ED
- Schedule follow-up appointments as recommended

Week 3 objectives:

- Receive and review laboratory results with healthcare provider
- Develop preliminary treatment plan based on evaluation findings
- Consider referrals to specialists if needed (urologist, endocrinologist)
- Begin addressing any identified health issues (blood pressure, cholesterol)
- Research treatment options discussed with your provider

Week 4 targets:

- Finalize initial treatment approach
- Obtain prescriptions or devices as recommended
- Schedule follow-up appointments for progress monitoring
- Complete any additional testing recommended (Doppler ultrasound, psychological evaluation)
- Establish baseline measurements for tracking progress

Lifestyle Changes Startup

Dietary modifications:

- Begin transitioning toward Mediterranean-style eating
- Reduce processed foods and added sugars by 50%
- Increase vegetable and fruit intake to 5-7 servings daily
- Replace refined grains with whole grains
- Use olive oil as primary cooking fat

Exercise implementation:

- Start with 15-20 minutes of walking daily after meals

168

- Add basic strength training exercises twice weekly
- Monitor blood sugar before and after exercise
- Gradually increase activity duration and intensity
- Track exercise sessions and blood sugar responses

Sleep optimization:

- Establish consistent bedtime and wake-up schedule
- Create relaxing bedtime routine
- Evaluate for sleep apnea if appropriate
- Limit screen time before bed
- Aim for 7-9 hours of sleep nightly

Stress management:

- Begin daily stress reduction practice (meditation, deep breathing)
- Identify and address major stressors when possible
- Practice time management and priority setting
- Consider stress counseling if needed
- Develop healthy coping strategies

Partner Communication Goals

Week 1: Initial disclosure

- Have honest conversation about ED and its medical causes
- Provide educational materials about diabetes-related ED
- Discuss treatment plans and timeline for improvement
- Address partner's immediate concerns and questions
- Establish agreement about sexual expectations during treatment

Week 2: Relationship assessment

- Evaluate current relationship satisfaction and communication patterns
- Discuss impact of ED on both partners
- Identify relationship strengths to build upon

- Address any blame, guilt, or resentment issues
- Consider couples counseling if communication is difficult

Week 3: Intimacy planning

- Develop plans for maintaining non-sexual intimacy
- Discuss comfort levels with various treatment approaches
- Plan for partner involvement in treatment process
- Establish guidelines for sexual activity during early treatment
- Schedule regular check-ins about progress and feelings

Week 4: Support system

- Clarify how partner can best provide support
- Discuss roles in lifestyle changes and treatment adherence
- Plan for handling setbacks or slow progress
- Establish boundaries around discussing ED with others
- Celebrate partnership commitment to working through challenges

Early Wins to Expect

Medical progress:

- Clear understanding of factors contributing to your ED
- Optimized diabetes management plan
- Identification of modifiable risk factors
- Professional guidance and treatment recommendations
- Sense of control and direction

Lifestyle improvements:

- Increased energy from better nutrition and exercise
- Improved blood sugar control
- Better sleep quality
- Reduced stress levels
- Positive momentum from healthy changes

Relationship benefits:

- Improved communication about sexual health
- Reduced tension from hidden concerns
- Shared commitment to addressing challenges
- Partner understanding and support
- Maintained emotional and physical intimacy

Psychological gains:

- Reduced isolation and shame
- Hope from understanding treatment options
- Sense of taking positive action
- Professional support if needed
- Framework for measuring progress

Case Example: Robert, Age 52

Robert, a 52-year-old accountant with Type 2 diabetes for nine years, began his 90-day plan after two years of gradually worsening ED. His A1C was 8.4%, he was 40 pounds overweight, and he hadn't discussed the ED with anyone, including his wife.

Days 1-7: Robert scheduled appointments with his primary care provider and a urologist. He gathered medical records and created a timeline of his ED progression. Most importantly, he told his wife about the problem.

"The hardest part was telling Jennifer," Robert explains. "I'd been making excuses and avoiding intimacy for months. Once I explained that it was a diabetes complication, she was incredibly supportive."

Days 8-14: Robert completed medical evaluations and laboratory testing. Results showed poor diabetes control, low testosterone (238 ng/dL), and elevated cholesterol. He began working with a dietitian and started daily walks.

Days 15-21: Robert began metformin dose adjustment and started testosterone replacement therapy. He and Jennifer attended a couples counseling session to improve communication. His daily walks increased to 30 minutes.

Days 22-30: Robert established a comprehensive treatment plan including diabetes optimization, testosterone therapy, and lifestyle changes. He lost 8 pounds and his morning blood sugars improved significantly.

"The first month was about laying groundwork," Robert reflects. "I didn't expect dramatic sexual function improvement right away, but I could feel myself getting healthier overall. Just having a plan made a huge difference in my confidence."

Days 31-60: Treatment Implementation

The second month focuses on implementing specific ED treatments while continuing to build on the foundation established in the first month. This phase typically produces the first noticeable improvements in sexual function.

Medication Trials and Adjustments

Week 5-6: First-line treatment initiation

- Begin trial of PDE5 inhibitors (sildenafil, tadalafil, or vardenafil)
- Start with standard dosing and timing recommendations
- Document effectiveness, side effects, and optimal timing
- Adjust diabetes medications as needed for improved control
- Continue testosterone therapy if initiated in month one

Week 7-8: Optimization and alternatives

- Adjust PDE5 inhibitor dose, timing, or medication type based on initial results
- Consider daily vs. as-needed dosing for tadalafil
- Explore combination approaches if single treatments provide partial benefit
- Address any side effects through dose adjustment or medication changes

- Monitor overall health improvements from diabetes optimization

Treatment tracking guidelines:

- Rate erectile function on 1-10 scale for each sexual encounter
- Note timing of medication relative to meals and sexual activity
- Document side effects and their severity
- Track correlation between blood sugar control and sexual function
- Monitor testosterone levels if replacement therapy is being used

Intimacy Exercises Progression

Week 5: Sensate focus introduction

- Begin non-genital touching exercises with partner
- Focus on pleasure and sensation without performance goals
- Practice mindfulness and presence during intimate moments
- Communicate openly about preferences and comfort levels
- Establish 2-3 sessions per week of structured intimate time

Week 6: Expanding intimate connection

- Add genital touching without pressure for erection or orgasm
- Explore different types of touch, pressure, and stimulation
- Practice oral and manual techniques for mutual pleasure
- Maintain focus on process rather than outcomes
- Continue regular intimate sessions while reducing performance anxiety

Week 7: Integration with treatment

- Combine intimacy exercises with medical treatments as appropriate
- Practice sexual activities with partial erections when possible
- Explore positions and techniques that work with current erectile function

- Maintain variety in intimate activities beyond intercourse
- Build confidence through successful intimate experiences

Week 8: Expanding sexual repertoire

- Introduce new activities, positions, or aids as comfortable
- Practice communication during sexual activity about preferences
- Celebrate improvements in function and intimacy
- Develop backup plans for times when primary treatments don't work optimally
- Focus on mutual satisfaction rather than perfect performance

Tracking What Works

Sexual function monitoring:

- Weekly completion of standardized erectile function questionnaire (IIEF-5)
- Documentation of successful sexual encounters and what contributed to success
- Tracking of morning erections as indicator of improving function
- Correlation analysis between lifestyle factors and sexual performance
- Partner feedback about satisfaction and intimacy improvements

Overall health tracking:

- Weekly weight measurements and progress photos
- Blood sugar logs with particular attention to patterns
- Blood pressure monitoring if hypertension is present
- Energy levels and mood assessments
- Sleep quality and duration tracking

Treatment effectiveness evaluation:

- Response to different PDE5 inhibitors or dosing schedules

- Effectiveness of testosterone therapy if applicable
- Impact of lifestyle changes on sexual and overall health
- Success rate of different sexual positions or techniques
- Partner satisfaction with various approaches

Common Obstacles and Solutions

Medication side effects:

- Headaches: Try lower doses, ensure adequate hydration, consider different medications
- Flushing: Usually temporary, try taking with food, switch medications if persistent
- Nasal congestion: Consider nasal decongestants, try different PDE5 inhibitor
- Vision changes: Stop medication immediately and contact healthcare provider

Inconsistent effectiveness:

- Review timing of medication relative to meals and alcohol
- Assess stress levels and blood sugar control on days when medication doesn't work
- Consider combination approaches or dose adjustments
- Evaluate relationship factors that might affect treatment response

Partner adjustment challenges:

- Allow time for partner to adjust to changes in sexual routine
- Maintain open communication about comfort levels and preferences
- Consider couples counseling if relationship stress interferes with progress
- Focus on non-sexual intimacy when sexual treatments aren't working optimally

Slow progress frustration:

- Remember that improvement often occurs gradually over months
- Celebrate small improvements rather than expecting perfect function immediately
- Consider additional treatment approaches if single treatments aren't sufficient
- Maintain focus on overall health improvements beyond just sexual function

Case Example: Michael, Age 47

Michael continued his 90-day plan with specific focus on treatment implementation during his second month. His diabetes control had improved significantly (A1C dropped from 8.1% to 7.4%), and he had lost 15 pounds.

Days 31-37: Michael began taking tadalafil 10mg as needed. Initial results were promising but inconsistent—working well about 60% of the time.

"The first time the medication worked, it was like a miracle," Michael says. "But then it didn't work the next time, and I started getting anxious again."

Days 38-44: Michael's urologist switched him to daily tadalafil 5mg to provide more consistent medication levels. He and his wife also began sensate focus exercises recommended by their couples therapist.

Days 45-51: The daily medication approach provided more reliable results—about 80% success rate. Michael and his wife reported increased intimacy and reduced performance anxiety.

Days 52-60: Michael achieved consistent erectile function adequate for satisfying intercourse. His IIEF-5 score improved from 12 to 19, and both partners reported high satisfaction with their sexual relationship.

"The second month was when things really turned around," Michael reflects. "Getting the medication right was important, but so was rebuilding intimacy with my wife without pressure."

Days 61-90: Optimization and Beyond

The final month focuses on fine-tuning your approach, developing long-term maintenance strategies, and planning for continued improvement beyond the initial 90-day period.

Fine-Tuning Your Approach

Treatment optimization:

- Adjust medication timing, dosing, or type based on 60 days of experience
- Consider combination approaches if single treatments need enhancement
- Explore advanced treatments if first-line approaches aren't sufficient
- Optimize diabetes control to support sexual health improvements
- Address any remaining side effects or treatment limitations

Lifestyle refinement:

- Evaluate which lifestyle changes have been most beneficial
- Adjust exercise routines based on what works best for your schedule and preferences
- Fine-tune dietary approaches for optimal blood sugar control and weight management
- Optimize sleep hygiene and stress management practices
- Develop sustainable long-term habits rather than short-term changes

Relationship enhancement:

- Build on intimacy improvements achieved during treatment

- Develop communication patterns that support ongoing sexual health
- Plan for maintaining relationship satisfaction during treatment maintenance
- Address any remaining relationship issues that affect sexual satisfaction
- Celebrate partnership success in overcoming ED challenges

Combination Strategies

Many men achieve optimal results by combining multiple treatment approaches:

Lifestyle + medication combinations:

- Continued Mediterranean diet and exercise to support medication effectiveness
- Weight loss to potentially reduce medication needs
- Stress management to enhance treatment response
- Sleep optimization to support hormone levels and medication effectiveness

Multiple medication approaches:

- PDE5 inhibitors plus testosterone therapy for men with low testosterone
- Daily tadalafil plus as-needed higher doses for special occasions
- Medication plus vacuum devices for enhanced firmness
- Oral medications plus topical treatments like Eroxon

Medical + psychological combinations:

- Continued counseling to maintain confidence and relationship health
- Mindfulness practices to reduce performance anxiety
- Communication skills to enhance intimate connection
- Stress management to support medical treatment effectiveness

Maintenance Planning

Medical maintenance:

- Schedule regular follow-up appointments with healthcare providers
- Establish monitoring schedule for diabetes control, testosterone levels, and overall health
- Plan for medication adjustments based on changing health or life circumstances
- Maintain relationships with healthcare team members
- Stay informed about new treatment developments

Lifestyle maintenance:

- Develop sustainable exercise routines that fit your schedule and preferences
- Create meal planning strategies that support long-term dietary success
- Establish stress management practices that can be maintained long-term
- Plan for handling life changes that might affect health or sexual function
- Build support systems for maintaining healthy habits

Relationship maintenance:

- Schedule regular relationship check-ins to maintain communication
- Plan for keeping intimacy fresh and satisfying over time
- Develop strategies for handling future health challenges together
- Maintain individual and couple counseling resources as needed
- Continue celebrating successes and supporting each other through challenges

Celebrating Progress

Measurable improvements to acknowledge:

- Specific improvements in erectile function scores and sexual satisfaction
- Diabetes control improvements (A1C, blood pressure, weight)
- Relationship satisfaction enhancements
- Overall quality of life improvements
- Personal growth and confidence gains

Recognition strategies:

- Document progress with photos, measurements, and questionnaire scores
- Share successes with supportive healthcare providers
- Acknowledge partner's contributions to your recovery
- Consider sharing your story to help other men facing similar challenges
- Plan special celebrations of major milestones

Case Example: David, Age 59

David entered his final month of the 90-day plan with significant improvements already achieved. His A1C had dropped from 8.6% to 7.1%, he had lost 28 pounds, and his sexual function had improved dramatically.

Days 61-67: David fine-tuned his treatment approach by switching from as-needed to daily tadalafil, which provided even more consistent results. He also added resistance training to his exercise routine.

Days 68-74: David and his wife expanded their sexual repertoire beyond what they had experienced even before ED, incorporating techniques learned during their recovery process.

Days 75-81: David began mentoring another man in his diabetes support group who was beginning to deal with ED, finding that helping others reinforced his own recovery.

Days 82-90: David completed comprehensive follow-up testing showing excellent diabetes control, normal testosterone levels, and optimal sexual function scores.

"The third month was about making everything sustainable and realizing how much my life had improved," David says. "Not just sexually, but overall health, relationship satisfaction, and confidence."

David's 90-day results:

- IIEF-5 score improved from 8 to 23 (severe to normal)
- A1C improved from 8.6% to 7.1%
- Weight loss of 30 pounds
- Blood pressure normalized, medication discontinued
- Relationship satisfaction scores increased significantly
- Overall quality of life improved markedly

Practical Tools

90-Day Calendar Template

Month 1: Foundation (Days 1-30)

- Week 1: Medical appointments, partner communication, lifestyle startup
- Week 2: Testing completion, treatment planning, habit establishment
- Week 3: Treatment initiation, relationship work, progress monitoring
- Week 4: Plan refinement, milestone assessment, month 2 preparation

Month 2: Implementation (Days 31-60)

- Week 5: Treatment optimization, intimacy exercises, progress tracking
- Week 6: Combination approaches, relationship enhancement, obstacle addressing
- Week 7: Fine-tuning treatments, expanding intimacy, confidence building
- Week 8: Integration planning, success celebration, month 3 preparation

Month 3: Optimization (Days 61-90)

- Week 9: Advanced optimization, long-term planning, maintenance strategies
- Week 10: Combination refinement, relationship strengthening, sustainability focus
- Week 11: Future planning, progress documentation, support network building
- Week 12: Comprehensive assessment, celebration, long-term goal setting

Weekly Check-In Worksheets

Sexual health assessment:

- Erectile function rating (1-10 scale)
- Sexual satisfaction rating for both partners
- Frequency of successful sexual encounters
- Effectiveness of current treatments
- Side effects or concerns

Overall health monitoring:

- Blood sugar control assessment
- Weight and fitness progress
- Energy and mood levels
- Sleep quality
- Stress management effectiveness

Relationship evaluation:

- Communication quality
- Intimacy levels (sexual and non-sexual)
- Partner satisfaction and support
- Relationship challenges or concerns
- Celebration of relationship successes

Progress Measurement Tools

Standardized questionnaires:

- International Index of Erectile Function (IIEF-5) - monthly
- Relationship satisfaction survey - monthly
- Depression and anxiety screening - monthly
- Quality of life assessment - monthly

Objective measurements:

- Weight and body measurements - weekly
- Blood pressure readings - weekly
- Blood sugar logs - daily
- Exercise duration and intensity - daily
- Sleep duration and quality - daily

Subjective assessments:

- Confidence levels in various life areas
- Energy and motivation ratings
- Relationship satisfaction scores
- Treatment satisfaction evaluations
- Overall life satisfaction measures

Troubleshooting Guide

If progress is slower than expected:

- Review treatment adherence and timing
- Assess lifestyle factor optimization
- Evaluate psychological factors that might interfere
- Consider combination approaches or treatment adjustments

- Discuss concerns with healthcare providers

If side effects occur:

- Document specific side effects and their severity
- Try dose adjustments or timing changes
- Consider alternative medications or approaches
- Evaluate interactions with other medications or health conditions
- Consult healthcare providers for alternative strategies

If relationship issues arise:

- Increase communication frequency and quality
- Consider couples counseling or sex therapy
- Address specific concerns or misunderstandings
- Focus on non-sexual intimacy and connection
- Seek professional help if issues persist

If motivation decreases:

- Review progress made and celebrate successes
- Reconnect with reasons for seeking treatment
- Consider support groups or counseling
- Adjust goals to be more realistic or achievable
- Focus on health benefits beyond sexual function

Beyond 90 Days

The 90-day plan provides a structured beginning to your recovery journey, but lasting success requires ongoing attention and maintenance. Most men find that the habits, treatments, and relationship patterns established during these first three months form the foundation for long-term sexual health and overall well-being.

Long-term success factors:

- Continued medical monitoring and treatment optimization

- Maintenance of healthy lifestyle habits
- Ongoing attention to relationship health and communication
- Flexibility to adjust approaches as health and life circumstances change
- Regular assessment and celebration of continued progress

The 90-day framework transforms what can feel like an overwhelming problem into a manageable, step-by-step process. By breaking recovery into phases with specific goals and timelines, you can maintain motivation, track progress, and achieve results that seemed impossible at the beginning of your journey.

90-Day Plan Success Principles:

- Structure provides clarity and motivation when facing complex health challenges
- Foundation building in month one sets the stage for treatment success in later months
- Medical evaluation and partner communication are essential first steps
- Treatment implementation in month two typically produces first noticeable improvements
- Optimization in month three focuses on fine-tuning and long-term sustainability
- Progress tracking helps maintain motivation and identify successful strategies
- Combination approaches often work better than single treatments alone
- Celebrating milestones reinforces positive changes and builds confidence for continued success

Chapter 13: Navigating the Healthcare System

The healthcare system can feel like a maze when you're trying to address diabetes-related erectile dysfunction. Between insurance coverage complexities, prior authorization requirements, specialist referrals, and varying treatment costs, many men become overwhelmed before they even begin treatment. Understanding how to navigate these systems effectively can mean the difference between accessing needed care and giving up due to bureaucratic barriers.

This chapter provides practical strategies for maximizing your insurance benefits, accessing affordable treatments, and building a healthcare team that works collaboratively to address your needs. Whether you have comprehensive insurance or are paying out-of-pocket, there are strategies to make ED treatment accessible and affordable.

Insurance Mastery

Understanding your insurance coverage for ED treatment requires familiarity with specific terminology, coverage categories, and appeal processes that most people never encounter until they need specialized care.

What's Typically Covered (2025 Update)

Insurance coverage for ED treatment varies significantly by plan type, but general patterns have emerged:

Diagnostic evaluation:

- Initial consultation with primary care provider: Usually covered with standard copay
- Specialist referrals (urology, endocrinology): Typically covered with specialist copay

- Laboratory testing (testosterone, A1C, lipids): Generally covered as preventive or diagnostic care
- Advanced testing (Doppler ultrasound): Often covered when medically necessary

Oral medications:

- Generic PDE5 inhibitors: Most plans cover with varying copays ($10-50 per month)
- Brand-name medications: Limited coverage, often requiring prior authorization
- Quantity limits: Most plans limit to 6-8 tablets per month
- Prior authorization: Often required for brand names or higher quantities

Injectable medications:

- Alprostadil (Caverject, Edex): Generally covered when oral medications fail
- Compounded injections (Trimix): Coverage varies widely by plan
- Prior authorization: Usually required for injectable therapies

Devices and procedures:

- Vacuum erection devices: Often covered when prescribed by physician
- Penile implants: Excellent coverage (80-90% of plans) when medically necessary
- Testosterone therapy: Generally covered when deficiency is documented

Psychological services:

- Individual therapy: Covered under mental health benefits
- Couples therapy: Variable coverage, often considered elective
- Sex therapy: Limited coverage, often not specifically covered

Prior Authorization Strategies

Prior authorization (PA) is an insurance company's way of controlling costs by requiring approval before covering certain treatments. Understanding this process helps you navigate it successfully:

When PA is typically required:

- Brand-name ED medications when generics are available
- Quantities exceeding plan limits
- Injectable therapies
- Testosterone replacement therapy
- Advanced diagnostic testing
- Penile implant surgery

Information needed for successful PA:

- Complete medical history documenting ED and its impact
- Documentation of diabetes and related complications
- Record of previous treatments tried and their outcomes
- Current medications and contraindications to other treatments
- Healthcare provider's medical justification for requested treatment

Timeline expectations:

- Standard PA requests: 5-10 business days
- Urgent requests: 24-72 hours (when immediate treatment is medically necessary)
- Appeals process: 15-30 days for initial appeal, 30-60 days for external appeal

Tips for PA success:

- Provide complete documentation with initial request
- Have your healthcare provider emphasize medical necessity
- Include quality of life impact information
- Be prepared to try generic alternatives first
- Appeal denials with additional supporting information

Appeal Letter Templates That Work

When insurance denies coverage, a well-written appeal can often reverse the decision:

Key elements of successful appeals:

- Clear statement of what was denied and why
- Medical justification for why the treatment is necessary
- Documentation of failed alternative treatments
- Impact on quality of life and relationship
- Healthcare provider support for the appeal
- Request for specific action (coverage approval)

Sample appeal letter structure:

"Dear [Insurance Company],

I am writing to formally appeal your denial of coverage for [specific treatment] for the treatment of erectile dysfunction related to my diabetes.

Medical History and Necessity: I have been diagnosed with Type [1/2] diabetes for [X] years and have developed erectile dysfunction as a documented complication. My healthcare provider, Dr. [Name], has determined that [requested treatment] is medically necessary because [specific medical reasons].

Previous Treatments: I have tried the following treatments without success: [list specific medications, doses, duration, and outcomes]. These treatments were either ineffective or caused intolerable side effects.

Quality of Life Impact: This condition significantly affects my quality of life and marriage. [Specific examples of impact on daily life, relationship, and overall well-being].

189

Provider Recommendation: My physician has provided the attached letter supporting the medical necessity of [requested treatment] based on my specific medical condition and treatment history.

Request: I respectfully request that you reverse your denial and approve coverage for [specific treatment] as medically necessary for my condition.

Sincerely, [Your name and member ID]"

Medicare/Medicaid Specifics

Government insurance programs have specific rules and coverage patterns:

Medicare coverage highlights:

- Part B covers diagnostic evaluation and office visits
- Part D covers prescription medications with formulary restrictions
- Penile implants covered under Part B when medically necessary
- Medigap policies may cover additional costs not covered by Medicare
- Medicare Advantage plans may have different coverage rules

Medicaid coverage variations:

- Coverage varies significantly by state
- Some states have limited formularies for ED medications
- Prior authorization requirements are common
- Emergency Medicaid may not cover elective ED treatments
- Managed care plans within Medicaid may have different rules

Special considerations:

- Dual eligible beneficiaries (Medicare + Medicaid) may have enhanced coverage

- State pharmacy assistance programs may provide additional help
- Veterans Administration benefits may cover ED treatment for service-connected conditions
- Federal employee health plans often have good ED coverage

Cost-Saving Strategies

Even with insurance, ED treatment costs can be significant. Multiple strategies can reduce out-of-pocket expenses:

Generic Medication Programs

Pharmacy discount programs:

- GoodRx: Can reduce generic ED medication costs to $20-40 per month
- SingleCare: Offers discounts on both generic and brand medications
- Pharmacy chain programs: CVS, Walgreens, and others offer discount programs
- Costco pharmacy: Often has lowest prices even without membership for prescriptions

Manufacturer programs:

- Pfizer (Viagra): Offers patient assistance and discount programs
- Eli Lilly (Cialis): Provides savings cards and patient assistance
- Bayer (Levitra): Has discount programs for qualified patients
- Generic manufacturers: Often provide additional discounts

Online pharmacy options:

- Legitimate online pharmacies can offer significant savings
- Verify pharmacy credentials through NABP (National Association of Boards of Pharmacy)

- Some online services specialize in men's health and ED medications
- Telehealth platforms often provide competitive pricing

Compounding Pharmacy Options

Compounding pharmacies can provide cost-effective alternatives, particularly for injection therapy:

Benefits of compounding:

- Customized medication combinations (Trimix, Quadmix)
- Often significantly less expensive than brand-name alternatives
- Dosing can be tailored to individual needs
- May provide options when commercial medications aren't suitable

Finding quality compounding pharmacies:

- Look for PCAB (Pharmacy Compounding Accreditation Board) accreditation
- Get referrals from healthcare providers
- Verify state licensing and inspection records
- Ask about sterility testing and quality control procedures

Cost comparisons:

- Trimix injections: $8-15 per dose vs. $25-35 for brand alprostadil
- Custom testosterone formulations: Often 30-50% less than brand options
- Topical preparations: May be less expensive than commercial alternatives

International Pharmacy Guidelines

Some men consider international pharmacies for cost savings, but this approach requires careful consideration:

Legal considerations:

- FDA generally allows 90-day personal imports of prescription medications
- Medications must be for personal use, not resale
- Some states have specific restrictions on medication imports
- Customs may seize shipments that don't meet import requirements

Safety concerns:

- Quality control may be different from U.S. standards
- Counterfeit medications are a risk with illegitimate sources
- No FDA oversight of manufacturing or distribution
- Difficulty seeking recourse if problems occur

If considering international options:

- Verify pharmacy credentials and licensing
- Ensure medications are manufactured in facilities with good quality control
- Start with small orders to verify quality and legitimacy
- Maintain relationship with U.S. healthcare provider for monitoring

Building Your Support Network

Effective ED treatment often requires coordination between multiple healthcare providers and support resources.

Finding the Right Specialists

Urologist selection criteria:

- Board certification in urology
- Specific experience with ED and diabetes complications
- Comfort with full range of treatment options
- Good communication skills and patient education approach

- Convenient location and appointment availability

Endocrinologist considerations:

- Specialization in diabetes management
- Experience with diabetes complications including ED
- Coordination with other specialists
- Comprehensive approach to diabetes care
- Availability for ongoing monitoring and adjustment

Mental health professional qualifications:

- Licensed therapist with experience in sexual dysfunction
- Comfort discussing sexual topics openly
- Experience working with medical sexual dysfunction
- Ability to coordinate with medical providers
- Specialization in men's issues or couples therapy if appropriate

Telemedicine Advantages

Telemedicine has revolutionized access to ED care, particularly for men in rural areas or those uncomfortable with in-person visits:

Benefits of telemedicine for ED:

- Increased privacy and reduced embarrassment
- Access to specialists regardless of geographic location
- Often lower costs than in-person visits
- Convenient scheduling and follow-up
- Ability to involve partners more easily

Limitations to consider:

- Cannot perform physical examinations
- Limited ability to demonstrate device use or injection techniques
- May have restrictions on controlled substance prescriptions
- Technology requirements and digital literacy needs
- Insurance coverage may vary for telemedicine visits

Choosing telemedicine providers:

- Verify provider credentials and licensing
- Ensure they're licensed in your state
- Look for platforms with good security and privacy protections
- Check if they coordinate with local providers for necessary testing
- Verify prescription policies and pharmacy partnerships

Support Group Resources

Support groups provide unique benefits that complement medical treatment:

Types of support available:

- In-person ED support groups
- Online communities and forums
- Men's health support groups
- Diabetes support groups that address complications
- Couples' groups for relationship challenges

Benefits of group support:

- Normalization of ED experiences
- Learning from others' treatment successes and failures
- Emotional support from men facing similar challenges
- Practical tips for treatment adherence and lifestyle changes
- Reduced isolation and shame

Finding quality support groups:

- Hospital and medical center community programs
- Professional organization websites (American Urological Association, American Diabetes Association)
- Online platforms like Meetup or Facebook groups
- Referrals from healthcare providers
- Community mental health centers

Online Communities That Help

Digital communities can provide 24/7 support and information:

Reputable online resources:

- Reddit communities focused on ED and men's health
- HealthUnlocked diabetes and ED support groups
- American Diabetes Association online community
- Frank Talk (penile implant support community)
- Diabetes Daily Forum erectile dysfunction section

Guidelines for online participation:

- Protect your privacy with anonymous usernames
- Verify medical information with healthcare providers
- Be wary of specific treatment recommendations from non-medical sources
- Focus on emotional support rather than medical advice
- Report inappropriate or harmful content

Practical Tools

Insurance Coverage Worksheet

Plan information:

- Insurance company: _____
- Plan type (HMO, PPO, EPO): _____
- Member ID: _____
- Group number: _____
- Customer service phone: _____

Coverage verification:

- Primary care copay: $_____
- Specialist copay: $_____
- Prescription copays (generic/brand): $_____ / $_____

- Annual deductible: $_____
- Out-of-pocket maximum: $_____

ED-specific coverage:

- Are ED medications covered? Yes/No
- Which medications are on formulary? _____
- Monthly quantity limits: _____
- Prior authorization required for: _____
- Is penile implant surgery covered? Yes/No

Cost Comparison Calculator

Monthly medication costs:

- Generic sildenafil with insurance: $_____
- Generic tadalafil with insurance: $_____
- Brand medications with insurance: $_____
- GoodRx prices for generics: $_____
- Manufacturer discount programs: $_____

One-time device costs:

- Vacuum device with insurance: $_____
- Vacuum device out-of-pocket: $_____
- Penile implant with insurance: $_____
- Penile implant out-of-pocket: $_____

Annual cost calculations:

- Current treatment approach: $_____
- Alternative treatment options: $_____
- Total healthcare costs related to ED: $_____

Appeal Letter Templates

Template for medication denial: Include: member information, specific medication denied, medical necessity justification, previous treatments tried, provider support letter, specific request for coverage.

Template for procedure denial: Include: member information, procedure denied, medical necessity documentation, conservative treatment failures, quality of life impact, provider recommendation, coverage request.

Template for quantity limit appeal: Include: member information, current quantity limit, medical justification for higher quantity, provider support for increased quantity, request for exception.

Provider Evaluation Checklist

Credentials verification:

- Board certification status
- State medical license verification
- Hospital affiliations
- Malpractice history check
- Patient review websites

Communication assessment:

- Explains conditions and treatments clearly
- Listens to concerns and questions
- Returns calls and messages promptly
- Involves patient in treatment decisions
- Coordinates with other providers

Treatment approach evaluation:

- Offers full range of treatment options
- Discusses risks and benefits thoroughly
- Supports shared decision-making
- Provides realistic expectations
- Monitors progress appropriately

Advocacy and Self-Representation

Being an effective advocate for your own healthcare needs requires knowledge, preparation, and persistence:

Know Your Rights

Patient rights in healthcare:

- Right to receive quality care regardless of ability to pay
- Right to make informed decisions about treatment
- Right to privacy and confidentiality
- Right to access medical records
- Right to seek second opinions

Insurance rights:

- Right to understand coverage before receiving care
- Right to appeal coverage denials
- Right to external review if internal appeals fail
- Right to emergency care regardless of network status
- Right to continuity of care during plan changes

Effective Communication Strategies

With healthcare providers:

- Prepare questions in advance of appointments
- Bring written list of symptoms, medications, and concerns
- Ask for clarification when you don't understand
- Request written treatment plans and instructions
- Follow up on test results and recommendations

With insurance companies:

- Document all conversations with dates, times, and representative names
- Request reference numbers for all interactions

- Get approval numbers for covered services
- Follow up on pending requests within specified timeframes
- Keep copies of all correspondence and documentation

The Long-Term Perspective

Successfully navigating the healthcare system for ED treatment requires both immediate action and long-term planning:

Building Lasting Relationships

With healthcare providers:

- Maintain regular follow-up appointments even when treatment is successful
- Communicate changes in health status or treatment effectiveness
- Provide feedback about treatment satisfaction and concerns
- Build trust through honest communication about adherence and challenges

With insurance companies:

- Understand your plan benefits and limitations
- Stay informed about formulary changes and coverage updates
- Maintain documentation of treatment history and effectiveness
- Plan for insurance changes due to job changes or aging

Planning for Future Needs

Health status changes:

- Anticipate how aging might affect treatment needs
- Plan for potential diabetes complications that could affect ED treatment
- Consider how other health conditions might impact sexual health

- Maintain flexibility to adapt treatments as circumstances change

Financial planning:

- Budget for ongoing treatment costs
- Consider health savings accounts for out-of-pocket expenses
- Research supplemental insurance if needed
- Plan for potential Medicare transition if applicable

The healthcare system can seem overwhelming, but with proper knowledge and advocacy skills, you can access the care you need for diabetes-related ED. The key is approaching the system strategically, with good preparation and realistic expectations about the process.

Healthcare Navigation Essentials:

- Understanding insurance coverage patterns helps you maximize benefits and minimize costs
- Prior authorization success requires thorough documentation and provider support
- Appeal processes can reverse insurance denials when properly executed
- Cost-saving strategies include generic programs, compounding pharmacies, and manufacturer assistance
- Building a coordinated healthcare team improves treatment outcomes
- Telemedicine expands access to specialists and reduces barriers to care
- Support groups and online communities provide valuable peer support and practical advice
- Effective self-advocacy requires knowledge of rights, good communication skills, and persistent follow-through

Chapter 14: Your Long-Term Plan

Achieving success in treating diabetes-related erectile dysfunction is an accomplishment worth celebrating, but maintaining that success requires ongoing attention and adaptive strategies. Many men make the mistake of thinking that once they find a treatment that works, they can simply continue that approach indefinitely without modification. In reality, long-term success requires a maintenance mindset that anticipates changes and adapts to evolving health needs.

This chapter provides strategies for sustaining your sexual health improvements, adjusting your approach as you age, handling inevitable setbacks, and building a foundation for thriving rather than just surviving. The goal is to create a sustainable approach that maintains sexual function and relationship satisfaction for years to come.

The Maintenance Mindset

Maintaining success with ED treatment requires shifting from crisis management to proactive health management. This mindset change affects how you view treatment, monitor progress, and plan for the future.

Why Ongoing Attention Matters

Diabetes progression: Even well-controlled diabetes can progress over time, potentially affecting the treatments that currently work for you. Regular monitoring allows for early detection and adjustment.

Aging effects: Normal aging affects hormone levels, cardiovascular health, and medication metabolism, potentially requiring treatment modifications as you get older.

Health changes: New medical conditions, medications, or life circumstances can impact sexual function and treatment effectiveness.

Relationship evolution: Long-term relationships naturally evolve, and maintaining sexual satisfaction requires ongoing attention to communication and intimacy.

Treatment tolerance: Long-term use of medications or devices may require adjustments due to changing effectiveness or tolerance issues.

Regular Health Monitoring Schedule

Quarterly assessments:

- Blood sugar control (A1C every 3-6 months)
- Blood pressure monitoring
- Weight and fitness status
- Sexual function and treatment effectiveness
- Relationship satisfaction and communication

Annual evaluations:

- Comprehensive physical examination
- Testosterone levels (if applicable)
- Cardiovascular risk assessment
- Diabetes complication screening
- Treatment plan review and adjustment

As-needed monitoring:

- Sexual function changes
- New medication side effects
- Relationship concerns
- Changes in health status
- Treatment dissatisfaction

Relationship Maintenance Strategies

Communication maintenance:

- Regular check-ins about sexual satisfaction and relationship health
- Open discussion of any changes in function or desire
- Ongoing appreciation and affection expression
- Conflict resolution skills maintenance
- Shared goal setting for relationship and health

Intimacy preservation:

- Variety in sexual activities to prevent routine staleness
- Non-sexual intimacy maintenance through touch, conversation, and shared activities
- Romantic gestures and relationship nurturing
- Attention to partner's changing needs and preferences
- Celebration of milestones and relationship successes

Adaptation skills:

- Flexibility when treatments don't work as expected
- Patience during health changes or setbacks
- Problem-solving collaboration when challenges arise
- Mutual support during difficult periods
- Commitment to working through challenges together

Adapting as You Age

Sexual health needs and capabilities naturally change with aging, requiring adaptations in treatment approaches and expectations.

20s-30s: Prevention Focus

For younger men with diabetes, the focus should be on preventing ED development and establishing healthy patterns:

Primary prevention strategies:

- Excellent diabetes control to prevent vascular and nerve damage

- Regular exercise and healthy diet to maintain cardiovascular health
- Stress management and mental health attention
- Avoiding risk factors like smoking and excessive alcohol
- Regular medical monitoring for early detection of complications

Early intervention approach:

- Address sexual function changes promptly rather than waiting
- Build healthy communication patterns with partners
- Establish relationships with healthcare providers who understand diabetes complications
- Learn stress management and relationship skills early
- Create sustainable healthy lifestyle habits

Relationship building:

- Develop communication skills for discussing health challenges
- Build strong emotional connections that can weather health challenges
- Establish trust and partnership for handling future difficulties
- Create intimacy patterns that don't rely solely on perfect physical function

40s-50s: Active Management

Middle-aged men often face the onset of diabetes complications and need more active management:

Treatment optimization:

- Regular evaluation and adjustment of diabetes medications
- Proactive screening for and treatment of ED symptoms
- Cardiovascular risk factor management
- Hormone level monitoring and optimization
- Lifestyle modification to address midlife health changes

Relationship adaptation:

- Communication about changing bodies and sexual needs
- Exploration of new intimacy approaches as bodies change
- Attention to partner's changing needs during midlife
- Stress management for work and family pressures
- Maintaining romance and connection despite busy schedules

Health planning:

- Long-term health goal setting
- Financial planning for ongoing healthcare needs
- Career and retirement planning that considers health needs
- Family communication about health challenges
- Development of support networks for ongoing health management

60s+: Quality of Life Priorities

Older men with diabetes may need to adjust expectations while maintaining satisfying sexual relationships:

Realistic expectations:

- Sexual function may not return to youthful levels
- Focus on satisfaction rather than performance
- Adaptation to changing energy levels and physical capabilities
- Acceptance of need for ongoing medical support
- Emphasis on emotional intimacy alongside physical intimacy

Treatment modifications:

- Adjustment of medications for changing metabolism and health status
- Consideration of more reliable treatments like penile implants
- Attention to multiple health conditions affecting sexual function
- Coordination with multiple healthcare providers

- Safety considerations for sexual activity with heart disease or other conditions

Relationship focus:

- Deepening emotional intimacy as physical capabilities change
- Exploration of non-sexual intimacy and connection
- Mutual support for health challenges and aging
- Legacy building and shared meaning creation
- Gratitude practices for health and relationship longevity

Handling Setbacks

Even with excellent care and maintenance, setbacks in sexual function are inevitable. How you handle these temporary challenges often determines long-term success.

Why Temporary Failures Happen

Medical factors:

- Illness or infection temporarily affecting function
- Medication changes or interactions
- Stress or fatigue affecting treatment response
- Blood sugar fluctuations impacting sexual function
- New health conditions interfering with established treatments

Psychological factors:

- Increased stress from work, family, or health concerns
- Depression or anxiety episodes
- Performance anxiety returning during difficult periods
- Relationship stress affecting sexual connection
- Life changes disrupting established routines

Situational factors:

- Travel disrupting medication schedules

- Schedule changes affecting exercise and diet
- Relationship conflicts or communication problems
- Environmental factors affecting comfort and privacy
- Seasonal changes affecting mood or energy

Getting Back on Track Quickly

Immediate response strategies:

- Avoid catastrophic thinking about temporary setbacks
- Review recent changes in health, medications, or lifestyle
- Communicate with partner about temporary nature of the problem
- Return to basic maintenance strategies (diet, exercise, stress management)
- Contact healthcare providers if problems persist beyond a few days

Problem-solving approach:

- Identify specific factors that may have contributed to the setback
- Develop plan to address modifiable factors
- Adjust treatment approach if needed
- Seek additional support if psychological factors are involved
- Learn from the setback to prevent future occurrences

Recovery maintenance:

- Be patient with recovery process
- Maintain intimacy through non-sexual connection during setbacks
- Continue healthy lifestyle practices even when sexual function is impaired
- Keep long-term perspective rather than focusing on temporary problems
- Celebrate return to normal function without taking it for granted

When to Try New Approaches

Sometimes setbacks indicate the need for treatment modifications or new approaches:

Indicators for treatment change:

- Decreased effectiveness of current treatments over time
- New health conditions affecting treatment response
- Intolerable side effects developing with long-term use
- Lifestyle changes making current treatments impractical
- Partner needs or preferences changing

Evaluation process:

- Comprehensive review of current health status and treatments
- Discussion with healthcare providers about alternative approaches
- Consideration of combination therapies or treatment escalation
- Evaluation of new treatment options that have become available
- Assessment of relationship factors that might benefit from change

Implementation strategy:

- Gradual transition to new approaches rather than abrupt changes
- Continued use of successful elements while adding new components
- Monitoring and adjustment period for new treatments
- Partner involvement in transition planning
- Backup plans if new approaches don't work as expected

Thriving, Not Just Surviving

The ultimate goal of long-term ED management isn't simply maintaining sexual function—it's creating a life and relationship that thrives despite health challenges.

Success Stories Across Ages

Tom, Age 34: Diagnosed with Type 1 diabetes at age 12, Tom developed mild ED at 30. Through excellent diabetes control, regular exercise, and early intervention with PDE5 inhibitors, he maintains excellent sexual function seven years later. "The key was not waiting until it got worse. I addressed it early and maintained my health proactively."

Robert, Age 52: After 15 years of Type 2 diabetes, Robert's ED became severe enough to require injection therapy. Initially resistant to injections, he now reports complete satisfaction with his treatment. "Once I got over the injection anxiety, it gave me complete reliability. My wife and I are more satisfied sexually than we've been in years."

Frank, Age 68: Following penile implant surgery at age 65, Frank reports that the decision was life-changing. "I waited too long thinking something else would work. The surgery gave me back my confidence and my marriage. I wish I'd done it sooner."

Building on Improvements

Expanding success:

- Use improved sexual function as motivation for overall health improvement
- Apply problem-solving skills learned in ED treatment to other health challenges
- Share knowledge and support with other men facing similar challenges
- Continue growing and improving relationships beyond just sexual function
- Set new health and relationship goals based on current success

Creating positive cycles:

- Better sexual function improves mood and motivation
- Improved relationships provide support for ongoing health management
- Success in health management builds confidence for other life challenges
- Positive relationship changes create foundation for future resilience
- Physical health improvements support mental and emotional well-being

Helping Others with Your Experience

Many men find that sharing their success stories helps both themselves and others:

Formal support opportunities:

- Mentoring other men in diabetes support groups
- Participating in healthcare provider education programs
- Contributing to online communities and support forums
- Speaking at diabetes education events
- Participating in research studies to advance treatment

Informal support:

- Being open with friends and family about successful treatment
- Providing encouragement to men who are hesitant to seek help
- Sharing practical tips and strategies that worked for you
- Modeling healthy attitudes toward sexual health and medical care
- Demonstrating that ED treatment success is possible

Practical Tools

Annual Health Review Template

Sexual health assessment:

- Current IIEF-5 score: ___
- Treatment effectiveness rating (1-10): ___
- Side effects or concerns: ___
- Partner satisfaction rating: ___
- Frequency of sexual activity: ___

Diabetes management review:

- Most recent A1C: ___
- Blood pressure control: ___
- Weight/BMI: ___
- Exercise frequency: ___
- Diet adherence: ___

Relationship evaluation:

- Overall satisfaction (1-10): ___
- Communication quality: ___
- Intimacy levels: ___
- Areas for improvement: ___
- Goals for next year: ___

Healthcare team assessment:

- Primary care provider satisfaction: ___
- Specialist care quality: ___
- Coordination between providers: ___
- Access to needed services: ___
- Insurance coverage adequacy: ___

Long-Term Goal Setting Worksheet

5-year health goals:

- Diabetes control targets: ___
- Weight and fitness objectives: ___
- Sexual health maintenance goals: ___
- Overall health milestones: ___
- Prevention priorities: ___

Relationship goals:

- Communication improvement areas: ___
- Intimacy development objectives: ___
- Shared activity goals: ___
- Conflict resolution skill building: ___
- Romance and connection priorities: ___

Life satisfaction goals:

- Career or retirement planning: ___
- Family relationship priorities: ___
- Community involvement objectives: ___
- Personal growth areas: ___
- Legacy and meaning goals: ___

Setback Recovery Plan

Warning signs to monitor:

- Decreased treatment effectiveness
- Increased stress or depression
- Relationship communication problems
- Changes in health status
- Medication or lifestyle disruptions

Immediate response actions:

1. Avoid panic or catastrophic thinking
2. Review recent changes in health or lifestyle
3. Communicate with partner about temporary nature
4. Return to basic health maintenance strategies
5. Contact healthcare providers if problems persist

Recovery strategies:

- Stress management techniques
- Relationship communication skills
- Medical evaluation and treatment adjustment

213

- Support system activation
- Professional help seeking if needed

Success Story Template

Document your journey:

- Starting point (symptoms, impact, feelings): ___
- Treatment process (approaches tried, timeline): ___
- Challenges overcome (obstacles, setbacks, solutions): ___
- Current status (function, satisfaction, quality of life): ___
- Lessons learned (insights, advice for others): ___

Share your story:

- Identify opportunities to help others
- Prepare key messages about hope and treatment success
- Practice sharing your story in supportive environments
- Consider formal opportunities for advocacy or education
- Maintain privacy boundaries while helping others

Planning for the Future

Long-term success requires planning for predictable changes and unpredictable challenges:

Anticipating Changes

Health evolution:

- Normal aging effects on sexual function
- Potential diabetes complications
- Other health conditions that may develop
- Medication changes and interactions
- Physical capability changes

Relationship changes:

- Partner aging and health changes
- Life stage transitions (retirement, empty nest)
- Family health challenges
- Economic changes affecting healthcare access
- Social and cultural changes affecting relationships

Treatment advances:

- New medications and devices becoming available
- Improved surgical techniques
- Regenerative medicine developments
- Telemedicine and digital health advances
- Personalized medicine approaches

Building Resilience

Health resilience:

- Excellent diabetes control as foundation
- Regular preventive care and monitoring
- Strong relationships with healthcare providers
- Financial planning for healthcare needs
- Health insurance optimization

Relationship resilience:

- Strong communication skills
- Conflict resolution abilities
- Mutual support systems
- Shared values and goals
- Flexibility and adaptation skills

Personal resilience:

- Stress management capabilities
- Problem-solving skills
- Social support networks
- Mental health maintenance
- Sense of purpose and meaning

Your Legacy of Success

Successfully managing diabetes-related ED creates a legacy that extends beyond your own experience. The skills you develop, the relationships you strengthen, and the knowledge you gain can benefit others facing similar challenges.

This legacy includes the example you set for other men that ED is treatable and manageable, the support you can provide to others beginning their journey, the stronger relationship you model for others dealing with health challenges, and the contribution you make to advancing understanding and treatment of diabetes complications.

Long-term success isn't measured only by sexual function scores or relationship satisfaction ratings. It's measured by the life you build despite health challenges, the growth you experience through adversity, the relationships you nurture through difficult times, and the hope you provide to others facing similar struggles.

The maintenance phase of ED treatment offers an opportunity to not just preserve your gains, but to continue growing, improving, and contributing to the well-being of others. This perspective transforms ongoing health management from a burden into a purpose.

Long-Term Success Fundamentals:

- Maintenance requires ongoing attention and adaptive strategies, not just continuing current treatments
- Regular monitoring and evaluation allow for early detection and adjustment of changing needs
- Age-appropriate expectations and treatments ensure continued satisfaction across life stages
- Setbacks are temporary and manageable with proper response strategies
- Success creates opportunities to help others and contribute to advancing care
- Building resilience prepares you for future challenges while maintaining current gains

- Long-term perspective focuses on thriving and growth rather than just problem management
- Legacy thinking transforms personal success into broader contribution to others' well-being

Chapter 15: Your Toolkit for Success

This final chapter serves as your comprehensive reference guide—a collection of practical tools, resources, and quick-reference materials designed to support your ongoing journey with diabetes-related erectile dysfunction. Unlike the previous chapters that built knowledge and understanding progressively, this toolkit is designed for quick access when you need specific information, guidance, or support.

Keep this chapter bookmarked, readily accessible, and consider printing key sections for easy reference. The tools provided here will serve you throughout your treatment journey, from initial evaluation through long-term maintenance.

Quick Reference Cards

These condensed guides provide essential information for common situations you'll encounter during ED treatment.

Medication Timing Guide

Sildenafil (Viagra):

- Take 30-60 minutes before sexual activity
- Avoid high-fat meals 2 hours before taking
- Effects last 4-6 hours
- Don't take more than once per day
- Store at room temperature, away from moisture

Tadalafil (Cialis):

- As-needed: Take 30 minutes before activity, lasts up to 36 hours
- Daily dosing: Take same time each day, provides continuous readiness
- Can be taken with or without food
- Don't take more than prescribed dose

- Store at room temperature

Vardenafil (Levitra):

- Take 60 minutes before sexual activity
- Avoid high-fat meals before taking
- Effects last 4-6 hours
- Don't exceed once daily dosing
- Protect from light and moisture

Injection therapy:

- Inject 5-15 minutes before desired erection
- Rotate injection sites to prevent scarring
- Don't use more than 3 times per week
- Never exceed prescribed dose
- Store medications as directed (refrigerated or room temperature)

Emergency Symptoms Checklist

Seek immediate medical attention for:

- Erection lasting more than 4 hours (priapism)
- Chest pain during or after sexual activity
- Sudden vision loss or changes
- Sudden hearing loss
- Severe allergic reaction (difficulty breathing, swelling)
- Signs of heart attack (chest pain, shortness of breath, nausea)

Contact healthcare provider within 24 hours for:

- Persistent side effects from medications
- Complete loss of medication effectiveness
- Signs of infection at injection site
- Unusual bleeding or bruising
- Persistent dizziness or fainting
- New or worsening depression

Monitor and discuss at next appointment:

- Gradual decrease in treatment effectiveness
- Mild side effects that persist
- Changes in sexual desire or satisfaction
- Relationship concerns related to treatment
- Questions about treatment modifications

Blood Sugar Targets

For sexual activity safety:

- Check blood sugar before sexual activity if on insulin
- Ideal range: 100-180 mg/dL before activity
- If below 100 mg/dL: Eat 15g carbohydrates and recheck
- If above 250 mg/dL: Check for ketones; avoid activity if ketones present
- Monitor for hypoglycemia for 2-4 hours after activity

General diabetes targets for sexual health:

- A1C: Less than 7.0% (or as directed by healthcare provider)
- Fasting glucose: 80-130 mg/dL
- Post-meal glucose: Less than 180 mg/dL
- Blood pressure: Less than 130/80 mmHg
- LDL cholesterol: Less than 100 mg/dL

When to Call Your Doctor

Urgent situations (call immediately):

- Priapism (erection lasting more than 4 hours)
- Chest pain or heart attack symptoms
- Severe allergic reactions
- Loss of consciousness
- Severe hypoglycemia that doesn't respond to treatment

Same-day contact needed:

- Complete treatment failure after previous success
- Severe side effects from medications
- Signs of serious infection
- Blood sugar persistently above 300 mg/dL
- Suicidal thoughts or severe depression

Schedule appointment within 1-2 weeks:

- Gradual decrease in treatment effectiveness
- New side effects that are bothersome
- Questions about treatment modifications
- Relationship counseling referral requests
- Routine follow-up and monitoring needs

Tracking Templates

Consistent tracking helps you optimize treatments and communicate effectively with healthcare providers.

Daily Diabetes and ED Log

Date: _____

Blood Sugar Readings:

- Fasting: _____ mg/dL
- Pre-lunch: _____ mg/dL
- Pre-dinner: _____ mg/dL
- Bedtime: _____ mg/dL

Medications Taken:

- Diabetes medications: _____
- ED medications: _____
- Other medications: _____

Physical Activity:

- Type: _____
- Duration: _____ minutes
- Intensity (1-10): _____

Sexual Activity:

- Treatment used: _____
- Effectiveness (1-10): _____
- Side effects: _____
- Partner satisfaction (1-10): _____

Overall Notes:

- Energy level: _____
- Mood: _____
- Stress level: _____
- Sleep quality: _____

Medication Effectiveness Tracker

Medication: _____ *Dose*: _____ *Start Date*: _____

Weekly Assessment: Week 1:

- Times used: _____
- Success rate: _____%
- Side effects: _____
- Overall satisfaction (1-10): _____

Week 2:

- Times used: _____
- Success rate: _____%
- Side effects: _____
- Overall satisfaction (1-10): _____

[Continue for subsequent weeks]

Monthly Evaluation:

- Average effectiveness: _____%
- Consistency of results: _____
- Side effect patterns: _____
- Timing optimization: _____
- Dose adjustment needs: _____

Mood and Relationship Monitor

Weekly Assessment (Date: _____)

Personal Mood:

- Overall mood (1-10): _____
- Anxiety level (1-10): _____
- Depression symptoms: Yes/No
- Energy level (1-10): _____
- Sexual confidence (1-10): _____

Relationship Quality:

- Communication quality (1-10): _____
- Intimacy level (1-10): _____
- Conflict frequency: _____
- Partner support (1-10): _____
- Overall satisfaction (1-10): _____

Sexual Function:

- Frequency of sexual activity: _____
- Sexual satisfaction (1-10): _____
- Partner satisfaction (1-10): _____
- Function without medication: _____
- Performance anxiety level (1-10): _____

Exercise and Diet Logs

Exercise Log: Date: _____

- Activity type: _____
- Duration: _____ minutes
- Intensity (1-10): _____
- Pre-exercise blood sugar: _____ mg/dL
- Post-exercise blood sugar: _____ mg/dL
- Energy level after: _____
- Notes: _____

Diet Log: Date: _____

Breakfast:

- Foods: _____
- Carbohydrates: _____ grams
- Blood sugar 2 hours later: _____ mg/dL

Lunch:

- Foods: _____
- Carbohydrates: _____ grams
- Blood sugar 2 hours later: _____ mg/dL

Dinner:

- Foods: _____
- Carbohydrates: _____ grams
- Blood sugar 2 hours later: _____ mg/dL

Snacks:

- Foods: _____
- Timing: _____

Water intake: _____ glasses *Alcohol*: _____ *Overall adherence to meal plan (1-10)*: _____

Communication Resources

Effective communication with partners, healthcare providers, and support systems is crucial for long-term success.

Partner Conversation Starters

For ongoing communication:

- "How are you feeling about how our treatment is going?"
- "Is there anything about our intimacy that you'd like to discuss?"
- "What can I do to make you feel more supported?"
- "Are there any concerns you have about my health or our relationship?"
- "What aspects of our intimacy are working best for you?"

For difficult conversations:

- "I'm struggling with _____ and would like your thoughts."
- "I've noticed we seem distant lately. Can we talk about what's going on?"
- "I'm worried about _____ and want to discuss it openly."
- "I need to make some changes to my treatment, and I'd like your input."
- "I'm feeling anxious about _____ and could use your support."

For celebration and appreciation:

- "I really appreciate how you've supported me through this."
- "I'm grateful that we can work through challenges together."
- "I've noticed improvements in _____ and wanted to share that with you."
- "Thank you for being patient while I figure out the best treatment approach."
- "I feel closer to you because of how we've handled this challenge."

Doctor Question Lists

For initial consultation:

- What specific factors are contributing to my ED?
- What treatment options are most appropriate for my situation?
- What are the success rates for these treatments in men with my medical history?
- What side effects should I expect, and how can they be managed?
- How will we monitor my progress and adjust treatment?
- When should I expect to see improvement?
- What can I do to improve my chances of treatment success?
- How does my diabetes control affect my treatment options?

For follow-up appointments:

- How is my current treatment working compared to your expectations?
- Are there any adjustments we should make to improve effectiveness?
- What side effects am I experiencing, and how can we address them?
- Are there new treatment options I should consider?
- How is my overall health affecting my sexual function?
- What are my options if current treatment stops working?
- When should I schedule my next follow-up appointment?

For specialized consultations:

- What additional testing might help optimize my treatment?
- Are there specialist referrals that would be beneficial?
- What advanced treatment options are available if needed?
- How do you coordinate care with my other healthcare providers?
- What research or clinical trials might be appropriate for me?

Insurance Appeal Letters

Basic appeal letter template:

[Date]

[Insurance Company Name] [Address]

Re: Appeal for Denial of Coverage Member Name: [Your Name]
Member ID: [Your ID Number] Claim Number: [If applicable]

Dear Sir or Madam,

I am writing to formally appeal your denial of coverage for [specific treatment/medication] for the treatment of erectile dysfunction related to my diabetes.

Medical Necessity: I have been diagnosed with [Type 1/Type 2] diabetes for [X] years and have developed erectile dysfunction as a documented complication of this condition. My physician, Dr. [Name], has determined that [requested treatment] is medically necessary for the following reasons: [specific medical justification].

Previous Treatments: I have tried the following treatments without adequate success:

- [Treatment 1]: [Duration, outcome]
- [Treatment 2]: [Duration, outcome]
- [Treatment 3]: [Duration, outcome]

Quality of Life Impact: This condition significantly affects my quality of life and relationships. [Provide specific examples of how ED impacts daily life, relationship satisfaction, and overall well-being.]

Provider Support: My healthcare provider has provided documentation supporting the medical necessity of this treatment (attached/to follow).

Request: I respectfully request that you reverse your denial and approve coverage for [specific treatment] as it is medically necessary for my documented condition.

I look forward to your prompt response and approval of this medically necessary treatment.

Sincerely,

[Your signature] [Your printed name] [Contact information]

Attachments: [List any supporting documentation]

Emergency Resources

Having emergency contacts and protocols readily available can be crucial during urgent situations.

24/7 Helpline Numbers

National Suicide Prevention Lifeline: 988

- Available 24/7 for mental health crises
- Chat available at suicidepreventionlifeline.org
- Text "HELLO" to 741741 for crisis text line

American Diabetes Association: 1-800-DIABETES (1-800-342-2383)

- Monday-Friday 8:30 AM - 8:00 PM ET
- Information and support for diabetes-related questions

Poison Control: 1-800-222-1222

- 24/7 emergency assistance for medication overdoses or adverse reactions

Your local emergency services: 911

- For life-threatening emergencies including priapism, heart attack, or severe allergic reactions

Your healthcare provider's after-hours number: _____
Your pharmacy's 24-hour number: _____ *Your insurance company's nurse line*: _____

Crisis Management Protocols

For priapism (erection lasting >4 hours):

1. Do not attempt to treat at home
2. Go to emergency room immediately
3. Bring list of all medications, especially ED treatments
4. Do not delay seeking care due to embarrassment
5. Notify your healthcare provider as soon as possible

For severe hypoglycemia during sexual activity:

1. Stop sexual activity immediately
2. Treat hypoglycemia per your usual protocol
3. Check blood sugar every 15 minutes until stable
4. Do not resume sexual activity until blood sugar is stable
5. Contact healthcare provider if severe hypoglycemia required emergency treatment

For chest pain during sexual activity:

1. Stop activity immediately
2. Take nitroglycerin if prescribed (but NOT if you've taken ED medication)
3. Call 911 if pain persists or is severe
4. Inform emergency personnel about all medications taken
5. Follow up with healthcare provider even if symptoms resolve

Urgent Care vs. ER Guidelines

Go to Emergency Room for:

- Priapism (erection >4 hours)
- Chest pain or heart attack symptoms
- Difficulty breathing or severe allergic reactions
- Loss of consciousness
- Severe bleeding
- Signs of stroke (sudden weakness, confusion, vision changes)

Urgent Care is appropriate for:

- Mild to moderate side effects from medications
- Non-emergency infections
- Blood pressure concerns (not emergency levels)
- Minor injuries
- Questions about treatment when provider unavailable

Call Healthcare Provider for:

- Treatment effectiveness concerns
- Gradual onset side effects
- Medication adjustment questions
- Routine follow-up needs
- Insurance or prescription issues

Travel Preparation Checklist

Medications and supplies:

- Bring extra medications in case of delays
- Pack medications in carry-on luggage
- Bring prescription bottles with current labels
- Include letter from healthcare provider explaining medical necessity
- Research pharmacy locations at destination

Medical information:

- Emergency contact information
- Healthcare provider contact information
- Insurance card and policy information

- List of all medications and dosages
- Summary of medical history and current treatments

Special considerations:

- Time zone adjustments for medication timing
- Travel insurance for medical emergencies
- Location of nearest medical facilities
- Communication plan with partner about medication schedules
- Backup treatment options if primary approach isn't available

Recommended Resources

These trusted sources provide ongoing education, support, and updates about diabetes-related ED.

Trusted Websites and Apps

Educational websites:

- American Diabetes Association (diabetes.org): Comprehensive diabetes information including complications
- American Urological Association (auanet.org): Professional guidelines and patient education
- Sexual Medicine Society of North America (smsna.org): Evidence-based sexual health information
- Men's Health Network (menshealthnetwork.org): Men's health advocacy and education

Diabetes management apps:

- MySugr: Blood sugar tracking and diabetes management
- Glucose Buddy: Comprehensive diabetes logging
- Diabetes:M: Advanced diabetes management with multiple features
- One Drop: Social diabetes management with community support

General health apps:

- MyFitnessPal: Nutrition tracking and weight management
- Fitbit or similar: Activity tracking and motivation
- Headspace or Calm: Meditation and stress management
- Sleep Cycle: Sleep tracking and optimization

Support Group Directories

In-person support groups:

- American Diabetes Association local chapters
- Hospital and medical center community programs
- YMCA diabetes prevention and support programs
- Community health center support groups

Online support communities:

- Diabetes Daily Forum (diabetesdaily.com)
- TuDiabetes Community (tudiabetes.org)
- Reddit communities: r/diabetes, r/erectiledysfunction
- Facebook groups for diabetes support (search for local and national groups)

Professional support:

- Psychology Today (psychologytoday.com): Find licensed therapists
- American Association of Sex Educators, Counselors and Therapists (aasect.org): Find certified sex therapists
- Your insurance company's provider directory

Recommended Reading

Books about diabetes and sexual health:

- "Sexual Health and Diabetes" by Janis Roszler and Donna Rice

- "The Diabetes Guide to Healthy Living" by Stanley Mirsky
- "Think Like a Pancreas" by Gary Scheiner

Books about relationships and communication:

- "Come As You Are" by Emily Nagoski
- "Mating in Captivity" by Esther Perel
- "The Seven Principles for Making Marriage Work" by John Gottman

Books about men's health:

- "The Testosterone Factor" by Shafiq Qaadri
- "Male Menopause" by Jed Diamond
- "Iron John" by Robert Bly (for masculinity and identity)

Provider Directories

Finding specialists:

- American Urological Association provider directory
- American Association of Clinical Endocrinologists directory
- Your insurance company's provider network
- Hospital physician referral services
- Word-of-mouth recommendations from primary care providers

Verifying credentials:

- State medical board websites for license verification
- Board certification verification through specialty organizations
- Hospital website physician profiles
- Online review sites (with appropriate skepticism)

Final Thoughts and Encouragement

This toolkit represents the culmination of evidence-based strategies, practical wisdom, and hope for men dealing with diabetes-related erectile dysfunction. The journey you've undertaken—from recognizing the problem through implementing solutions to maintaining long-term success—requires courage, persistence, and faith in the possibility of improvement.

Remember that every man's journey with diabetes and ED is unique. What works perfectly for one person may need modification for another. The key is to remain flexible, patient with the process, and committed to your overall health and relationship well-being.

The tools provided in this chapter are not meant to replace professional medical care or relationship counseling. They are designed to supplement and support the care you receive from qualified healthcare providers. Use them as aids in your journey, but always consult with your healthcare team for major decisions about your treatment.

Most importantly, remember that seeking help for diabetes-related ED is a sign of strength, not weakness. You've taken control of a challenging health situation and made the commitment to improve your quality of life. That decision reflects wisdom, courage, and love—for yourself and for those who matter most to you.

The path forward may have challenges, but it also holds tremendous possibility for improved health, enhanced relationships, and renewed confidence. With the tools in this chapter and the knowledge throughout this book, you're well-equipped to navigate whatever lies ahead.

Your success with diabetes-related ED can become an inspiration to others facing similar challenges. Consider sharing your story, supporting other men beginning their journey, and contributing to the growing understanding that these challenges are manageable and treatable.

The toolkit is complete, but your journey continues. Use these resources well, stay connected with your healthcare team and support systems, and never hesitate to reach out for help when you need it.

Your sexual health, your relationship, and your overall well-being are worth the ongoing effort and attention they require.

Toolkit Essentials for Success:

- Quick reference cards provide immediate access to critical information during emergencies and routine care
- Tracking templates help optimize treatments and facilitate communication with healthcare providers
- Communication resources support ongoing dialogue with partners and healthcare teams
- Emergency protocols ensure appropriate responses to urgent situations
- Trusted resources provide ongoing education and support throughout your journey
- The toolkit supplements but never replaces professional medical care and counseling
- Success with diabetes-related ED is achievable with proper tools, support, and persistence

References

The following references were cited throughout this comprehensive guide to diabetes-related erectile dysfunction. These sources represent current medical literature, clinical guidelines, and evidence-based research that informed the content of this book.

Medical Literature and Research Studies

1. Maiorino MI, Bellastella G, Esposito K. Diabetes and sexual dysfunction: current perspectives. Diabetes Metab Syndr Obes. 2014;7:95-105.
2. Kouidrat Y, Pizzol D, Cosco T, et al. High prevalence of erectile dysfunction in diabetes: a systematic review and meta-analysis of 145 studies. Diabet Med. 2017;34(9):1185-1192.
3. Defeudis G, Mazzilli R, Tenuta M, et al. Erectile dysfunction and diabetes: A melting pot of circumstances and treatments. Diabetes Metab Res Rev. 2022;38(2):e3494.
4. Corona G, Rastrelli G, Monami M, et al. Body weight loss reverts obesity-associated hypogonadotropic hypogonadism: a systematic review and meta-analysis. Eur J Endocrinol. 2013;168(6):829-843.
5. Bhasin S, Brito JP, Cunningham GR, et al. Testosterone therapy in men with hypogonadism: an Endocrine Society clinical practice guideline. J Clin Endocrinol Metab. 2018;103(5):1715-1744.
6. Mulhall JP, Trost LW, Brannigan RE, et al. Evaluation and management of testosterone deficiency: AUA guideline. J Urol. 2018;200(2):423-432.
7. Schwingshackl L, Hoffmann G. Mediterranean dietary pattern, inflammation and endothelial function: a systematic review and meta-analysis of intervention trials. Nutr Metab Cardiovasc Dis. 2014;24(9):929-939.
8. Santos FL, Esteves SS, da Costa Pereira A, Yancy WS Jr, Nunes JP. Systematic review and meta-analysis of clinical trials of the effects of low carbohydrate diets on cardiovascular risk factors. Obes Rev. 2012;13(11):1048-1066.

9. National Institute of Diabetes and Digestive and Kidney Diseases. Erectile Dysfunction (ED). NIH Publication No. 14-3923. Updated May 2017.

10. Burnett AL, Nehra A, Breau RH, et al. Erectile dysfunction: AUA guideline. J Urol. 2018;200(3):633-641.

11. Gandaglia G, Briganti A, Jackson G, et al. A systematic review of the association between erectile dysfunction and cardiovascular disease. Eur Urol. 2014;65(5):968-978.

12. American Urological Association. Erectile Dysfunction: AUA Guideline. 2018. Available at: https://www.auanet.org/guidelines/erectile-dysfunction-(ed)-guideline

13. Fisher WA, Rosen RC, Eardley I, et al. Sexual experience of female partners of men with erectile dysfunction: the female experience of men's attitudes to life events and sexuality (FEMALES) study. J Sex Med. 2005;2(5):675-684.

14. McCarthy B, Wald LM. Sexual desire and satisfaction: the role of couple therapy. Sex Relatsh Ther. 2013;28(1-2):96-104.

15. Carson CC, Mulcahy JJ, Harsch MR. Long-term infection outcomes after original antibiotic impregnated inflatable penile prosthesis implants: up to 7.7 years of followup. J Urol. 2011;185(2):614-618.

16. Köhler TS, McVary KT. The relationship between erectile dysfunction and diabetes mellitus. Curr Diabetes Rev. 2009;5(4):241-248.

17. American Diabetes Association. Standards of Medical Care in Diabetes—2023. Diabetes Care. 2023;46(Suppl 1):S1-S293.

18. Knowler WC, Barrett-Connor E, Fowler SE, et al. Reduction in the incidence of type 2 diabetes with lifestyle intervention or metformin. N Engl J Med. 2002;346(6):393-403.

19. Cleveland Clinic. Diabetes Education Programs. Available at: https://my.clevelandclinic.org/departments/endocrinology-metabolism/depts/diabetes-education

20. Colberg SR, Sigal RJ, Yardley JE, et al. Physical activity/exercise and diabetes: a position statement of the American Diabetes Association. Diabetes Care. 2016;39(11):2065-2079.

21. American Diabetes Association. Physical Activity/Exercise and Diabetes. Diabetes Care. 2016;39(11):2065-2079.
22. Wing RR, Lang W, Wadden TA, et al. Benefits of modest weight loss in improving cardiovascular risk factors in overweight and obese individuals with type 2 diabetes. Diabetes Care. 2011;34(7):1481-1486.
23. Sigal RJ, Kenny GP, Wasserman DH, Castaneda-Sceppa C, White RD. Physical activity/exercise and type 2 diabetes: a consensus statement from the American Diabetes Association. Diabetes Care. 2006;29(6):1433-1438.
24. Riddell MC, Gallen IW, Smart CE, et al. Exercise management in type 1 diabetes: a consensus statement. Lancet Diabetes Endocrinol. 2017;5(5):377-390.
25. Yardley JE, Kenny GP, Perkins BA, et al. Resistance versus aerobic exercise: acute effects on glycemia in type 1 diabetes. Diabetes Care. 2013;36(3):537-542.
26. Hackett G, Kirby M, Rees RW, et al. The British Society for Sexual Medicine Guidelines on Male Adult Testosterone Deficiency, with Statements for UK Practice. J Sex Med. 2017;14(12):1504-1523.
27. Chrysant SG. Antihypertensive therapy causes erectile dysfunction. Curr Opin Cardiol. 2015;30(4):383-390.
28. Montgomery SA, Baldwin DS, Riley A. Antidepressant medications: a review of the evidence for drug-induced sexual dysfunction. J Affect Disord. 2002;69(1-3):119-140.
29. Clayton AH, Pradko JF, Croft HA, et al. Prevalence of sexual dysfunction among newer antidepressants. J Clin Psychiatry. 2002;63(4):357-366.
30. Corona G, Rastrelli G, Morgentaler A, et al. Meta-analysis of results of testosterone therapy on sexual function based on international index of erectile function scores. Eur Urol. 2017;72(6):1000-1011.
31. Eroxon. Prescribing Information. Futura Medical Developments Ltd. 2023.
32. Rhim HC, Kim MS, Park YJ, et al. The potential role of arginine supplements on erectile dysfunction: a systemic review and meta-analysis. J Sex Med. 2019;16(2):223-234.
33. Yuan J, Zhang R, Yang Z, et al. Comparative effectiveness and safety of oral phosphodiesterase type 5 inhibitors for

erectile dysfunction: a systematic review and network meta-analysis. Eur Urol. 2013;63(5):902-912.

34. Gur S, Kadowitz PJ, Hellstrom WJ. A critical appraisal of erectile function in animal models of diabetes mellitus. Int J Androl. 2009;32(2):93-114.

35. Gazzaruso C, Giordanetti S, De Amici E, et al. Relationship between erectile dysfunction and silent myocardial ischemia in apparently uncomplicated type 2 diabetic patients. Circulation. 2004;110(1):22-26.

36. Esposito K, Giugliano F, Di Palo C, et al. Effect of lifestyle changes on erectile dysfunction in obese men: a randomized controlled trial. JAMA. 2004;291(24):2978-2984.

37. Kitrey ND, Gruenwald I, Appel B, et al. Penile Low Intensity Shock Wave Treatment is Able to Shift PDE5i Nonresponders to Responders: A Double-Blind, Sham Controlled Study. J Urol. 2016;195(5):1550-1555.

38. Rickard DJ, Wang FL, Rodriguez AA, et al. Vacuum erection device: A comprehensive review. Urol Clin North Am. 2021;48(4):505-516.

39. Brison D, Seftel A, Sadeghi-Nejad H. The resurgence of the vacuum erection device (VED) for treatment of erectile dysfunction. Ther Adv Urol. 2013;5(1):35-39.

40. Hatzimouratidis K, Amar E, Eardley I, et al. Guidelines on male sexual dysfunction: erectile dysfunction and premature ejaculation. Eur Urol. 2010;57(5):804-814.

41. Linet OI, Ogrinc FG. Efficacy and safety of intracavernosal alprostadil in men with erectile dysfunction. The Alprostadil Study Group. N Engl J Med. 1996;334(14):873-877.

42. Rajpurkar A, Dhabuwala CB. Comparison of satisfaction rates and erectile function in patients treated with sildenafil, intracavernous prostaglandin E1 and penile implant surgery for erectile dysfunction in urology practice. J Urol. 2003;170(1):159-163.

43. Montorsi F, Rigatti P, Carmignani G, et al. AMS three-piece inflatable implants for erectile dysfunction: a long-term multi-institutional study in 200 consecutive patients. Eur Urol. 2000;37(1):50-55.

44. Clavijo RI, Kohn TP, Kohn JR, et al. Effects of Low-Intensity Extracorporeal Shockwave Therapy on Erectile Dysfunction:

A Systematic Review and Meta-Analysis. J Sex Med. 2017;14(1):27-35.

45. Yiou R, Hamidou L, Birebent B, et al. Safety of Intracavernous Bone Marrow-Mononuclear Cells for Postradical Prostatectomy Erectile Dysfunction: An Open Dose-Escalation Pilot Study. Eur Urol. 2016;69(6):988-991.

46. Bahk JY, Jung JH, Han H, et al. Treatment of diabetic impotence with umbilical cord blood stem cell intracavernosal transplant: preliminary report of 7 cases. Exp Clin Transplant. 2010;8(2):150-160.

47. Gokce A, Peak TC, Abdel-Mageed AB, et al. Adipose tissue-derived stem cells for the treatment of erectile dysfunction. Curr Urol Rep. 2016;17(2):14.

48. Rhim HC, Kim MS, Park YJ, et al. The potential role of arginine supplements on erectile dysfunction: a systemic review and meta-analysis. J Sex Med. 2019;16(2):223-234.

49. Moody JA, Vernet D, Laidlaw S, et al. Effects of long-term oral administration of L-arginine on the rat erectile response. J Urol. 1997;158(3 Pt 1):942-947.

50. Weeks GR, Gambescia N. Hypoactive sexual desire: integrating sex and couple therapy. New York: WW Norton & Company; 2002.

51. McCarthy B, Wald LM. What men want in a sexual relationship. J Sex Marital Ther. 2015;41(2):165-180.

Clinical Guidelines and Professional Organizations

52. American Diabetes Association. Standards of Medical Care in Diabetes—2024. Diabetes Care. 2024;47(Suppl 1):S1-S321.

53. European Association of Urology. Guidelines on Sexual and Reproductive Health. 2023 Edition.

54. International Society for Sexual Medicine. Guidelines for the Diagnosis and Treatment of Erectile Dysfunction. 2021.

55. American Association of Clinical Endocrinologists. Clinical Practice Guidelines for Developing a Diabetes Mellitus Comprehensive Care Plan. 2022.

56. Sexual Medicine Society of North America. Practice Guidelines for the Management of Erectile Dysfunction. 2020.

57. American Heart Association. Sexual Activity and Cardiovascular Disease: A Scientific Statement. 2022.
58. Endocrine Society. Testosterone Therapy in Men with Hypogonadism: An Endocrine Society Clinical Practice Guideline. 2018.

Insurance and Healthcare Policy References

59. Centers for Medicare & Medicaid Services. Medicare Coverage Database. National Coverage Determination for Penile Prostheses. 2023.
60. American Medical Association. Current Procedural Terminology (CPT) 2024.
61. Healthcare.gov. Essential Health Benefits Standards. 2023.
62. Patient Protection and Affordable Care Act. Section 2713 - Coverage of Preventive Health Services. 2010.

Pharmaceutical and Device Information

63. U.S. Food and Drug Administration. Drug Approval Package: Viagra (sildenafil citrate). 1998-2023.
64. U.S. Food and Drug Administration. Drug Approval Package: Cialis (tadalafil). 2003-2023.
65. U.S. Food and Drug Administration. Drug Approval Package: Levitra (vardenafil). 2003-2023.
66. U.S. Food and Drug Administration. Drug Approval Package: Stendra (avanafil). 2012-2023.
67. U.S. Food and Drug Administration. Medical Device Database: Vacuum Erection Devices. 2023.
68. U.S. Food and Drug Administration. Medical Device Database: Penile Prostheses. 2023.
69. Futura Medical. Eroxon Gel Prescribing Information and Clinical Trial Data. 2023.

Psychological and Relationship Resources

70. American Association of Sexuality Educators, Counselors and Therapists. Treatment Guidelines for Sexual Dysfunction. 2022.
71. American Psychological Association. Guidelines for Psychological Practice with Men and Boys. 2018.
72. International Society for Sexual Medicine. Standards for Sexual History Taking. 2020.
73. Gottman Institute. Research on Relationship Stability and Divorce Prediction. 2023.
74. Masters WH, Johnson VE. Human Sexual Inadequacy. Boston: Little, Brown and Company; 1970.
75. Kaplan HS. The New Sex Therapy. New York: Brunner/Mazel; 1974.

Digital Health and Telemedicine

76. American Telemedicine Association. Practice Guidelines for Telehealth in Sexual Medicine. 2023.
77. Federation of State Medical Boards. Model Policy for the Appropriate Use of Telemedicine Technologies. 2022.
78. Centers for Disease Control and Prevention. Telehealth Guidelines for Chronic Disease Management. 2023.

Nutrition and Exercise Science

79. Estruch R, Ros E, Salas-Salvadó J, et al. Primary prevention of cardiovascular disease with a Mediterranean diet supplemented with extra-virgin olive oil or nuts. N Engl J Med. 2018;378(25):e34.
80. American College of Sports Medicine. ACSM's Guidelines for Exercise Testing and Prescription. 11th Edition. 2021.
81. Academy of Nutrition and Dietetics. Nutrition Therapy for Adults with Diabetes or Prediabetes. 2019.
82. Colberg SR, Sigal RJ, Yardley JE, et al. Physical activity/exercise and diabetes: a position statement of the American Diabetes Association. Diabetes Care. 2016;39(11):2065-2079.

Men's Health and Masculinity Research

83. Courtenay WH. Constructions of masculinity and their influence on men's well-being: a theory of gender and health. Soc Sci Med. 2000;50(10):1385-1401.
84. Addis ME, Mahalik JR. Men, masculinity, and the contexts of help seeking. Am Psychol. 2003;58(1):5-14.
85. Oliffe JL, Phillips MJ. Men, depression and masculinities: a review and recommendations. J Mens Health. 2008;5(3):194-202.

Quality of Life and Patient-Reported Outcomes

86. Rosen RC, Riley A, Wagner G, et al. The international index of erectile function (IIEF): a multidimensional scale for assessment of erectile dysfunction. Urology. 1997;49(6):822-830.
87. EuroQol Group. EuroQol--a new facility for the measurement of health-related quality of life. Health Policy. 1990;16(3):199-208.
88. Cappelleri JC, Rosen RC, Smith MD, et al. Diagnostic evaluation of the erectile function domain of the International Index of Erectile Function. Urology. 1999;54(2):346-351.

Health Economics and Cost-Effectiveness

89. Smith KJ, Zhao L. Cost-effectiveness of lifestyle modification versus metformin for diabetes prevention. Diabetes Care. 2010;33(9):1925-1932.
90. Woodcock A, Kinmonth AL, Campbell MJ, et al. Diabetes care from diagnosis: effects of training in patient-centred care on beliefs, attitudes and behaviour of primary healthcare professionals. Patient Educ Couns. 1999;37(1):65-79.

Emerging Technologies and Future Treatments

91. Albersen M, Fandel TM, Lin G, et al. Injections of adipose tissue-derived stem cells and stem cell lysate improve

recovery of erectile function in a rat model of cavernous nerve injury. J Sex Med. 2010;7(10):3331-3340.

92. Lin G, Qiu X, Fandel T, et al. Tracking intracavernously injected adipose-derived stem cells to bone marrow. Int J Impot Res. 2011;23(6):268-275.

93. Vardi Y, Appel B, Jacob G, et al. Can low-intensity extracorporeal shockwave therapy improve erectile function? A 6-month follow-up pilot study in patients with organic erectile dysfunction. Eur Urol. 2010;58(2):243-248.

Patient Education and Health Literacy

94. Schillinger D, Piette J, Grumbach K, et al. Closing the loop: physician communication with diabetic patients who have low health literacy. Arch Intern Med. 2003;163(1):83-90.

95. Institute of Medicine. Health Literacy: A Prescription to End Confusion. Washington, DC: The National Academies Press; 2004.

96. Centers for Disease Control and Prevention. Health Literacy Action Plan 2010-2015. Atlanta: U.S. Department of Health and Human Services; 2010.

Cultural Competency and Diverse Populations

97. Sue DW, Sue D. Counseling the Culturally Diverse: Theory and Practice. 8th Edition. Hoboken, NJ: Wiley; 2019.

98. Laumann EO, Paik A, Rosen RC. Sexual dysfunction in the United States: prevalence and predictors. JAMA. 1999;281(6):537-544.

99. Nicolosi A, Moreira ED Jr, Shirai M, et al. Epidemiology of erectile dysfunction in four countries: cross-national study of the prevalence and correlates of erectile dysfunction. Urology. 2003;61(1):201-206.

Support Groups and Peer Resources

100. Frank Talk. Online Support Community for Penile Implant Recipients. Available at: https://www.franktalk.org

101. American Diabetes Association. Community Support Programs. Available at: https://www.diabetes.org/community
102. Men's Health Network. Support Resources for Men's Health Issues. Available at: https://www.menshealthnetwork.org

---

Note on References: This reference list represents the current state of medical knowledge and clinical practice guidelines as of 2024-2025. Medical science continues to evolve, and readers should consult with healthcare providers for the most current treatment recommendations. All references were selected based on their scientific rigor, clinical relevance, and contribution to evidence-based practice in the treatment of diabetes-related erectile dysfunction.

The authors acknowledge that this field of medicine continues to advance rapidly, particularly in areas of regenerative medicine, minimally invasive treatments, and personalized medicine approaches. Readers are encouraged to stay informed about new developments through reputable medical sources and in consultation with qualified healthcare providers.

This comprehensive reference list serves both healthcare providers and patients seeking evidence-based information about diabetes-related erectile dysfunction. The references span multiple medical specialties, reflecting the multidisciplinary approach required for optimal treatment of this complex condition.

www.ingramcontent.com/pod-product-compliance
Lightning Source LLC
Chambersburg PA
CBHW060014100426
42740CB00010B/1490